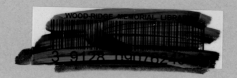

How We Do Family

How We Do Family

From Adoption to Trans Pregnancy, What We Learned About Love and LGBTQ Parenthood

TRYSTAN REESE

THE EXPERIMENT

NEW YORK

HOW WE DO FAMILY: *From Adoption to Trans Pregnancy, What We Learned About Love and LGBTQ Parenthood*
Copyright © 2021 by Trystan Reese

The Experiment, LLC
220 East 23rd Street, Suite 600
New York, NY 10001-4658
theexperimentpublishing.com

THE EXPERIMENT and its colophon are registered trademarks of The Experiment, LLC. Many of the designations used by manufacturers and sellers to distinguish their products are claimed as trademarks. Where those designations appear in this book and The Experiment was aware of a trademark claim, the designations have been capitalized.

The Experiment's books are available at special discounts when purchased in bulk for premiums and sales promotions as well as for fundraising or educational use. For details, contact us at info@theexperimentpublishing.com.

Library of Congress Cataloging-in-Publication Data available upon request

ISBN 978-1-61519-756-9
Ebook ISBN 978-1-61519-757-6

Jacket design by Beth Bugler
Cover photograph by Mark Pratt-Russum
Text design by Sarah Schneider
Author photograph by Rhys Harper
Photographs courtesy of the author unless otherwise noted.

Manufactured in the United States of America

First printing June 2021
10 9 8 7 6 5 4 3 2 1

To my parents, Janet and Clay, who taught me that you don't have to do anything special to become a parent. Just open the door and be ready when children walk in.

CONTENTS

CHAPTER ONE

HOW WE DO LOVE

———

Becoming a parent after only a year of dating was never the plan.

Biff and I had celebrated our first anniversary as boyfriends and had just moved in together. Our goal *had* been to take it slowly and date for at least a year before living together, but we broke that promise when my lease was up. We found a spacious one-bedroom on the top floor of the same Hollywood apartment building I was living in when we first met. We both adored the vintage wrought iron railings in the lobby, the creaky elevator, and the view overlooking a secret garden with a fountain and swinging bench. At that point in our relationship, our biggest disagreements had been over Biff's dog, Olive, who barked at anyone and everyone. Other than our differing approaches to doggy discipline, we just fit together. Where I was spontaneous and adventurous, he was thoughtful and frugal. We balanced each other out and had both come to depend on our relationship as our primary source of love and support.

Becoming a person who was open to that love wasn't as simple. I came out as transgender at age nineteen. I was living in Portland, Oregon, as a teenage girl, in a tormented relationship with a boy whose mood swings oscillated between weeks-long bouts of depression and regular fits of anger at the world. In retrospect, it was a deeply troubled relationship that I should have left long before I did, but I have grace for my younger self who didn't truly have any models for healthy non-heterosexual relationships.

One night it came to me with such precision and clarity that I knew it couldn't possibly be wrong: I'm a boy. I suddenly knew that I had never been a girl. Though the realization rang clear as a bell, it still took time to come to terms with my transgender identity. I went to meetups for transgender men and started performing as a drag king at an all-ages queer night club. The coming-out process was rocky: People who attend support groups are often those without much support to give. Many were confused by me—I was a girl who said I was a boy but still looked and sounded like a girl and was also attracted to other boys. Somehow, I still managed to barrel forward in my self-discovery.

EVEN WITHOUT ROLE models or access to formal language, I was clear about my gender identity (the internal knowledge I possessed about my own gender): I was a boy. I was also clear about my sexual orientation (who I was attracted to): I was a boy who liked other boys, which made me gay. "Oh, so you're actually a straight woman?" people would ask me. "Why would you want to be a man if you're just going to date other men anyway?" was also a common refrain. These inquiries sound quaint now, but to young adult me, they were confusing and devastating.

There was no confusion about my assigned sex, either: It was female ("born a woman," as we said then), but I was not at all clear about my gender expression (the ways in which one conveys their gender identity to the world). I knew I wasn't "butch," though I liked the snarling, leather-jacket-clad, motorcycle-driving, pompadour-sporting people I knew. I also couldn't be "femme," because others already viewed me as a girl, so when I put on makeup or a dress, I just looked like I was going to a high school dance. I was attracted to all kinds of boys, but none of them helped me discern who or what I was. I would have to do that for myself. I discovered that in order to continue on my journey, in order to keep living in this body, I would need to transition in one way or another.

Most of the people in my life told me I was delusional—that I wasn't *actually* transgender: I wasn't manly enough! I didn't date women! I didn't fit any of the criteria that would have designated me a Man. It took me three years to work up the nerve to see a doctor who could prescribe hormones legally, three years to begin the process of aligning my body to more accurately depict the person I knew myself to be. Once I started testosterone, my body began to slowly reconfigure itself into a new form, one that was slightly more muscular, slightly hairier, and with a slightly deeper voice (although none of those changes happened in the extremes I would have preferred). My ovulatory and menstrual processes were put on hold by the hormone shifts as well, and I even had to sign a legal form stating that I understood the fertility implications of testosterone. The paperwork inaccurately suggested that I may be rendered sterile by the hormonal transition process. It would be more than a decade before I would learn that my doctor had been misinformed about the actual impacts of testosterone on fertility. At the time, I was more than willing to sacrifice the possibility of future parenthood for the very real present reality of a more masculine appearance.

BEFORE MEETING AND FALLING IN LOVE with Biff at the end of my twenties, I worked my way through a cavalcade of disastrous romances. I had a lover who owned a series of gay bars throughout LA, and though he had slept with most of the go-go boys he employed, he decided that I had taken his virginity since I was the first (and only) person with a vagina he ever slept with. I dated a man who, even after six months of dating, refused to call me his boyfriend and then ghosted me completely in the middle of a trip to New York. One week later he was dating a different trans guy who was still in his teens. There was the dangerously handsome yet emotionally unstable graffiti artist who would skateboard to my apartment when he felt up to it then disappear for weeks on end, reemerging just long enough to hold my hand at a music festival, kiss me in front of strangers on the subway, then fade away once again.

I wasn't fixated on finding a forever partner, exactly. If you had asked me, I would have said I didn't have time for one. For work, I was a senior organizer at the National LGBTQ Task Force and was on the road eight months out of the year, following the anti-gay movement around the country, embedding myself in communities under attack, and teaching them how to talk to voters, raise money, and recruit volunteers. It was an advanced education in undoing bias, learning how to change people's minds one conversation at a time. I amassed thousands of data points that eventually made me a bias-busting ninja of sorts, with talking points for any argument at the ready. Coming home to my empty Hollywood apartment after these trips, I would wonder when love was going to happen to me. Many perfectly nice boys came and went, but none of them stayed.

Then one clear spring morning, I left my apartment to go to brunch at the home of my friends, a sweet couple named CT and Benji. As I came around their corner, I was distracted by a gorgeous boy heading right toward me.

"Hi!" I said.

He half-waved. "Are you going to the . . . thing? CT and Benji's thing?"

"Yeah! I'm Trystan."

"Hi." He nodded politely.

He had a nose ring and reddish-pink hair poking out from a black bandanna. He was wearing tight faded jeans that looked like they would be soft to the touch. Tall black boots. Steady blue eyes that carried an alluring mix of confidence, a don't-fuck-with-me vibe, and warmth. I suddenly found it hard to breathe. I tried to smile casually as I followed him into the courtyard and up the stairs of the yellow apartment building to brunch.

It was immediately clear that the food part of brunch wasn't happening anytime soon; someone had brought a whole coconut, and the guests were attempting to utilize a variety of scavenged tools to break it open. While others went to the porch to attempt a coconut/hacksaw maneuver, I sidled up to the boy I'd met outside. I learned that his name was Biff and that he ran a social group for gay, bi, trans, queer, and questioning men. He soon had an interested circle of listeners gathered around him, hanging on his every word.

"I want to come to your group!" a younger guy I didn't know blurted out. Others nodded in agreement as Biff took business cards out of his wallet and handed them around the circle. I had been trying to get a word in, to make my presence known, but wasn't able to break through the stream of conversation. By the time Biff got to me, he had run out of cards. He shrugged nonchalantly and said, "Sorry!" before moving on to a conversation about homeless issues in Downtown LA.

I couldn't figure out what was happening. Why couldn't I get his attention? Despite feeling like crap that morning, I had assembled a cute outfit (which was actually what I had worn to my side gig, bartending, the night before): striped vintage pants and suspenders over a black V-neck shirt. *What was I doing wrong?* This is not to say that I thought every gay man in the world would swoon over me, but a gay man around my age with an alternative sensibility was bound to at least notice me . . . right?

I went to the bathroom to gather myself and wash my hands. When I looked in the mirror and smiled, I saw it—a dark green piece of spinach from the salad I'd eaten just before walking out the door taking up an entire front tooth.

ARE YOU KIDDING ME??!!!

I was devastated and found myself near tears. *How do you come back from spinach in the teeth?*

I later found out that he thought it was a dead tooth that may have been indicative of a drug problem. Heart in my stomach, I stayed at the party as long as I could and left, humiliated. As I made the short walk home, I tried to forget about him.

Cue voice-over: "Trystan did not, in fact, forget about him."

INSTEAD, I FOUND HIM on Facebook, and the next time he posted about one of his meet-up groups, I went. It was in the back room of an LGBTQ church in West Hollywood, and I made sure to smile as much as possible so he would see how straight and white my teeth were. He warmed up to me eventually, and so began our flirtation. Well, I flirted with him and he tolerated it. This was not a dynamic I hated—it was actually a little fun. Then I learned he had a boyfriend, who was never around. I was undeterred, completely certain that I was a better catch than this boyfriend, whoever he was, and that I just had to convince Biff of this fact so he would leave (or cheat on) said boyfriend to be with me.

I had been with many men who had boyfriends, girlfriends, wives, or husbands. As a transgender man, it was hard enough for me to find men to date; I couldn't *also* require that they be emotionally—or actually—available. Predictably, these situations always ended in heartbreak. But old habits die hard, and I was hoping to finagle some kind of connection with Biff, boyfriend or no.

Over the following weeks we became friends, even hanging out after his group. I learned that he was from Bakersfield, which is both geographically and spiritually close to Lancaster, the California desert town where I grew up. I learned that he had been raised in a religious, conservative household and had fled as soon as he could, expecting LA to be a mecca of queer culture and support . . . only to find that queer "culture" mostly consisted of bars, and that queer "support" mostly consisted of online hookups.

Never one to let a dream die, Biff reached out to a friendly church and secured use of a spare room, free of charge, that he used to start his queer men's social group—a place for support and fraternity outside of the West Hollywood strip. He spent his days working at a homeless shelter, and at night would post about his group on Craigslist and Myspace. When he did go out dancing, he brought his handmade business cards with him, handing them out to anyone who looked lonely or in need of community. It was a motley crew that showed up each week: older men who reeked of desperation, younger men who were socially awkward, men of color who came in an attempt to flee the racism of the bar scene, and trans men who sought connection with other men who wouldn't judge them. And somehow, Biff held them all together.

I FELL IN LOVE with him almost immediately. He showed the same care and compassion to the man who brought him flowers but couldn't make eye contact that he showed to the PhD student who had just moved from Arkansas. Each week's meeting had a different theme (game night, discussion night, and so on), and he offered a social event each weekend (dim sum in Alhambra, hiking at Runyon Canyon, theater at the Pantages). He had seen a need for community and filled it, without ever getting paid or asking for anything in return. And everyone who came was welcomed the same.

One night, after a particularly rowdy and, I felt, infuriating game night in which no one was able to guess anyone's answers in charades, a few of us headed to The Standard rooftop bar in Downtown LA. I had a couple of drinks and was teasing Biff about polyamory. He had mentioned that he thought it was a good idea in theory, and I offered to help him put it into practice. The slight breeze lifted a chill off the hotel pool, and the hanging lights danced off his face. The Downtown LA skyline rose behind him as he sipped his cocktail, and I had never seen anyone so beautiful.

Eventually I left him with his friends and headed to the corner to catch a cab home. Later that night I received a text from him.

> So, I sense that there is an attraction between us, on your part at least. And I appreciate the attention, I really do. But I am in a relationship and I owe it to him to let that relationship play out. I ask that you respect that relationship and stop flirting with me entirely. Thanks.

My stomach sank. Had I made him uncomfortable? Had I ruined this? Why had I ignored the fact that he had a boyfriend? Was this why I was single—was there something wrong with me?

Then after the wave of shame, I felt something else . . . something new. Astonishment. Admiration. Awe. I had met a gay man in LA with principles. A gorgeous, smart, funny, passionate person who can assert a healthy boundary around his relationship.

Oh shit, I thought. *This is who you marry. The person who won't cheat* for *you won't cheat* on *you.*

When I received that text, I knew that what I did next could change the course of my life forever. I took a minute and composed an appropriately apologetic response:

Hey there! Thanks for bringing this up with me. I am so
sorry I've made you uncomfortable. Of course, I respect
your relationship, and will happily commit to being your
friend (without the flirting). Sorry again. See you soon.

I hit send and from that moment on, we were just friends.
I kept going to his group and kept inviting him to hangouts.
I never stopped being attracted to him, but I turned off the
flirt completely and worked to show him that I was capable of
listening and being respectful. I knew that one day he would
become available, and when he did I wanted him to think of
me as a solid prospect for a relationship. Then one day, a few
months later, a notification came up on my Facebook feed.

Biff Chaplow is now single.

I didn't think. I didn't ask my friends for advice. I didn't
hesitate. I just called him. When he answered, I asked simply,
"Hey, are you free tonight?" He said he was. "Do you want
to have dinner with me?" He said he did. "How about Geisha
House at eight?" He said yes and that night, we had our first
date.

I don't remember anything we said over dinner. I just
remember my nervousness and insecurity. He was so unlike
anyone I'd ever been with—would we be compatible? I tried to
imagine our bodies together and wasn't sure how it would work.
I guess some part of me had decided that only supermasculine
men would be interested in someone like me, who isn't exactly
feminine but whose body is more like the body of a feminine
person (I am slight in my frame, have almost no body hair,

11

and don't have the anatomy that most men associate with a masculine person). His demeanor was also different—he was direct and open. No games, no indecision.

He had just adopted a new puppy, Olive, and I had purchased some children's hair clips for her as a kind-of joke, but accidentally left them at my apartment.

"I'm sorry I forgot them! I'll bring them next time we hang out."

"Don't you live right around the corner? We can just go get them after dinner, right?"

I was mortified. I wasn't ready for him to come over, and forgetting the dog present had not been an attempt to get him to come to my apartment. I had genuinely just forgotten to bring them!

The shadow of past rejections loomed over me. "Gross." "Yuck." "Disgusting." "Come back when you have a dick." The echoes of gay male judgment haunted me, and I didn't feel strong enough to confront more. Not from him. Not that night. I wanted to have a few more dates before I had to face the reality of being transgender and trying to make it work with someone who was not. I wanted to live in the fantasy of a normal life for just a little longer.

But he was insistent, so we paid the bill and walked to my building. He sat on my bed in my studio apartment, and I couldn't breathe. We made awkward conversation as I located the purple barrettes and thrust them into his warm hands. I wanted to fall into his arms and tell him how long I had waited for this moment. But I just couldn't do it. I was too scared of what he might say or do, what I might find out about him. I stood up and reminded him that he had a train to catch. Confused, he said goodbye as I walked him out of my apartment and onto the street. As soon as he turned the corner, I realized how stupid I had been.

He was in your apartment! On your bed! That was your chance, you idiot!!!

I knew I needed more clarity about what this was so I could calibrate my expectations and level of fear and trepidation. I pulled out my phone and sent him a text.

> Hey, if you'd ever be up for a REAL date, I would be okay with that.

Not exactly the most up-front communication, but it was the best I could muster in the moment. I slowly walked back into my apartment building, slogged down the long hallway to my door, and let myself back in. It was another ten minutes before he resurfaced aboveground from the subway station by his Koreatown apartment. His text said:

> I would like that very much.

I let out the breath that it felt like I had been holding all evening, relieved that I hadn't ruined my chances, nor had I misread the situation. He *was* interested in me in *that* way. We went on our second date the following night; he made me fried plantains and black beans. He gave me flowers. Our first kiss was on the front steps of his apartment building, sun setting against the condos across the street, mouths sweet and sticky from the mango dessert. It was perfect.

THE NEXT YEAR was a whirlwind of being in love. In the early days we were committed to taking things slowly. Yes, we basically never left each other's sides and yes, we hardly ever spent a night apart, but we tried to be intentional about the stages of our relationship. We knew early on that we had something real, that it would take us somewhere special. We didn't want to rush it.

After one month of dating, I asked Biff to be my official "boyfriend." He said yes, and we talked about what that meant to both of us. We were ready to commit to a monogamous relationship, which meant (to us) that flirting with other people was fine, but kissing and anything beyond that were out of bounds.

At the time, many of our friends were rushing into "I love you" and "let's get married," and we didn't want to do that. We wanted to enjoy each stage of our relationship as it came, and looking back . . . I think that was a smart move on our part.

I hold so many moments within me from that time. Our first trip to the beach, which I had hoped would be romantic but was actually sandy and windy and cold. The first time we said, "I love you," which was at a party in San Francisco when we flew up there for Pride (I lost my ID somewhere in the club that night and had to travel back to LA without it, which meant intense scrutiny and a serious pat down at TSA that gave Biff a glimpse of how scary life as a trans person can actually be). Our first road trip, which took us all the way up the coast to visit my parents in Victoria, Canada (they both loved him right away). Despite the long drive, we didn't get sick of each other. Our first music festival, Coachella, where we saw The Postal Service and Lauryn Hill and slept in a tent baking in the hot sun all weekend long. The trip to Hawaii with my parents and sister—she and her boyfriend fought nonstop the whole time, and at one point we got lost with my dad on a hike. Biff somehow kept his cool and held my hand and forgave me for bringing all this chaos to his life. Soon I would understand that he was used to chaos, knew chaos intimately. His whole childhood had been a series of chaotic waves, and soon that torrent of chaos would stretch up from his early life and into our shared life, pulling us under its tow.

I HAD OCCASIONAL DREAMS of a baby. She had dark, liquid eyes and long eyelashes, and when I saw her in these dreams, I felt the deepest longing I had ever experienced. It was so clear to me—there was a baby who wanted to be born to us. But I chose not to say anything because I knew that the mention of a baby, so early on in a dating process, would indicate poor judgment. Those were the unspoken rules: You don't mention kids when you first start dating someone, and you *certainly* don't mention having a baby when you're a man dating another man! As a transgender person, I trained myself to tamp down any longings or behaviors that fell outside of the traditional gay male experience. I didn't want to challenge anyone's love for me, to test it. I was always afraid it would break.

I knew many transgender men who had given birth, but I had never considered doing it myself. As a young person, I had promised myself that I would never have children. It seemed like a thing that straight people did to give their lives more meaning. But then again, I had also planned to be a Broadway star, and that never happened. Once I met Biff, I realized that there was a whole other future I had never imagined for myself. When I looked at him, I could feel our entire lives stretching out before us . . . and those lives were intertwined, bound up with other possibilities I hadn't considered before.

I saw Biff with children all the time. We spent most weekends in Bakersfield visiting his family; his youngest sister, who was nineteen, had a toddler named Lucas. The little guy had a shaved head, which Biff told me was either to prevent lice or to emulate his mom's boyfriend, who was a skinhead. Lucas was quieter than any two-year-old I'd ever met before. I learned that he used to be more social before his mom started dating her new boyfriend, at which point Lucas stopped progressing and speaking. I couldn't believe how natural Biff was with Lucas. There was an easy grace about the two of them together—Biff understood Lucas's mangled attempts to communicate, could cheer him up when he scraped his knee, and was able to settle him down at the end of the night when he asked where his mommy was.

While in Bakersfield, we stayed with Biff's mom, Kimberley, and her husband Mark. Lucas stayed over too. Biff's sister had a hard time managing both a toddler and her boyfriend. Then she became pregnant again, and managing Lucas was harder than ever. We went up as often as we could, to help Biff's parents with Lucas. When Biff's sister went into labor with her second child, we took care of Lucas for several days in a row. The baby was named Hailey and soon after her birth, we spent weekends taking care of both kids.

Caring for children wasn't new to Biff; he had cared for his two younger siblings all the way through high school. And when Biff's sister wasn't getting along with their parents just after Lucas was born, Biff welcomed her and Lucas into his tiny studio apartment and became a 22-year-old gay boy who was taking care of his teenage sister and her newborn baby. He worked as a case manager at the shelter during the day and watched over infant Lucas in the evening and overnight.

It devastated him when his sister secretly started dating an older man who lived back in Bakersfield, and he was gutted when the man convinced her to move in with him and she quietly left LA, taking Lucas with her. Biff knew the situation wasn't going to be good for Lucas or his sister, but there was nothing he could do for either of them, other than support her by taking in Lucas and, once she was born, Hailey.

So, like I said . . . Biff was familiar with chaos. When we received a phone call from a social worker in September of 2011, letting Biff know that Lucas and Hailey were about to be removed from their home, Biff knew what he had to do—he would step in and care for these two small children for as long as they needed him. Biff had always been the glue that held his entire family together, and that role was about to be put to its greatest test. And I would have to decide whether I was willing to join him. If I was, it would mean becoming emergency parents to two toddlers I barely knew . . . and joining the chaos of his family forever.

Sure, we loved each other. But was that love enough to carry us through this crisis? We were both about to find out.

Notes from Life in Our Family

Understanding Trans Language

Though words shift all the time and are different across geography and between subsets of a community, as of the writing of this book, these are the Four Pillars of Identity that I use to undergird LGBTQ language:

ASSIGNED SEX AT BIRTH: what a doctor or midwife put on your birth certificate, usually based on visible external anatomy and sometimes informed by prenatal genetic testing. This is slowly shifting to become "sex traits": the many biological characteristics that exist inside each of us (chromosomal, anatomical, and hormonal). This category typically refers to your physical body and its characteristics. In our modern world, assigned sex at birth is typically male or female, although more states and provinces are adding a gender-neutral option on birth certificates.

Despite the relatively recent medical decision to make sex an either/or proposition, sex traits have always been diverse— many people contain a biological mix of "female" and "male" characteristics, such as: having a hormone imbalance (like polycystic ovarian syndrome); being born with medically ambiguous genitalia; experiencing gynecomastia (when a body that is otherwise considered male begins producing estrogen-based hormones, resulting in breast growth). People often believe that only our identities (our internal feeling about ourselves) exist on a spectrum, while nature contains only two rigid molds (male and female) from which our physical forms are cast. But that's simply not true; nature gifts each of us with the same biological clay that arranges itself into different versions of the same form. The biological form also exists on a spectrum! Most of us are on one end or the other of that spectrum, but there is so much in between those ends.

GENDER IDENTITY: our internal knowledge of our gender. Our gender identity usually develops in early childhood between ages three to five, but can sometimes come early and sometimes come late. Though most people develop this knowledge by kindergarten, I don't remember ever explicitly feeling like a boy *or* a girl. This, too, is a spectrum. There are boys and girls and men and women, and there are many other gender identities in between.

Throughout all of history people have existed who were not constrained by the ends of the spectrum, who know themselves to be, as the poet Nomy Lamm says, something in between, above, or beyond "man" or "woman." Those people have used many different words to describe themselves. During my lifetime, "genderqueer" and then "non-binary" have become the most common words used for this in the US and Canada. If one's gender identity is not in alignment with their assigned sex at birth—that is, if they are assigned female but know themselves to be a man—then they are "transgender." The prefix *trans-* means to cross over. If one's gender identity *is* in alignment with their assigned sex, they are considered "cisgender." The prefix *cis-* is Latin derived and is used in biology to describe something that is on the same side as another. Most people are cisgender. Most (though not all) non-binary people also consider themselves to be transgender, just as a rose may still be considered a flower.

GENDER EXPRESSION: the mix of gender cues we give the world, some of which we can control (such as our clothing choices and hairstyles) and some of which we can't (such as our height and the size of our hands). If one's gender expression is different from what is traditionally associated with their gender identity—such as a man who wears nail polish or a woman who wears suits—they may be considered "gender nonconforming."

SEXUAL ORIENTATION: who we are romantically and/or sexually attracted to. As a society, we pretty much understand that some people are attracted to their own gender (gay/lesbian), some are attracted to a gender other than their own (heterosexual/straight), and others are attracted to people across the gender spectrum (bisexual/pansexual). But if you go back fifty years or so, journalists regularly referred to bisexual people as predatory, mentally disturbed, and/or confused—essentially, bisexuality was treated then the same way that trans people are referred to now (in right-wing media, anyway). Even though biphobia (bias against bisexual people) still exists, the fact that we have evolved so much on bi issues inspires me to believe that perhaps we can also evolve on trans issues. To note: I haven't found any concrete data on this, but anecdotally, the word "bisexual" seems be falling out of favor of late, to be replaced by the word "pansexual," which many find more inclusive.

Your goal, when learning these concepts, should never be to know everything. It should be to know enough to be sensitive to others, to avoid ignorance, and to cultivate an attitude of humility that allows others to tell you when you've stepped out of line. As my mentor Beth Zemsky says, allyship is the ability to view the world through multiple lenses, and learning about those who are different from you is a great way to sharpen that lens.

CHAPTER TWO

HOW WE DO CRISIS

$\sim$

The drive north from LA to Bakersfield is only about ninety minutes, although this particular Friday afternoon, wondering if I was about to become a parent, it felt like an eternity. I stared at the checklist I'd made of all the things we needed to have on hand for Lucas and Hailey at our apartment to distract myself from the fear that something terrible might happen to them before we arrived.

I may have been aware of what we needed to do to get through the next few days, but I hadn't put any thought into (or perhaps was in denial of) what the situation meant for my relationship with Biff. I imagined that we would show the kids love, teach them how to say "please" and "thank you," read to them, keep them fed, and make sure they were clean, healthy, and happy. How hard could it be? Once we brought them to safety at our place, I figured their stay with us would be a fun adventure. Biff and I were great uncles, and I assumed that being a parent, whether temporary or permanent, wouldn't be all that different. It's rare to be called upon to step up in a way that will have a major positive impact on someone else's life. Agreeing to help Biff with his niece and nephew was *my* moment, and I was feeling the rush that sometimes accompanies doing the Right Thing.

Biff made his opinion clear as we made our way up the Grapevine toward Bakersfield. "Listen," he said, his voice somber. "I don't know if these kids are going to stay with us for a week, a month, a year, whatever. But this isn't something that we're going to do halfway. If you're in, that means you're all in. I'm not going to take these kids out of one unstable situation and drop them into another."

"I'm in," I promised.

"Yeah . . . I don't think you understand. What I'm saying is that if Hailey and Lucas end up needing a permanent home, then us taking them in now means you're also agreeing to be with me for the next eighteen years. Even if it isn't fun anymore. Even if you stop loving me. This is beyond even marriage, where divorce is an option. I'm saying you need to think about whether you're in this with me for the long haul."

I didn't need to think. "I'm in," I repeated. "I've been in since I first met you. You're my person." I tried to be reassuring, but I could tell he was wary. He didn't believe I knew what might be in store for us. Undeterred from my excitement about our adventure in parenting, I went back to checking off items on our to-do list and imagining our new life as caregivers.

We were still missing most basic supplies: a Pack 'n Play, sippy cups, pajamas, diapers. I'd sent a mass email to all of my LA parent friends asking them to pass along anything they had on hand that might be useful. We'd already scored a small car-shape bed for Lucas and set it up in a corner of our hastily rearranged living room before we left for Bakersfield. We figured we'd grab the remaining items from Target on the way back to LA and put it all on my credit card with our fingers crossed, hoping we didn't hit my limit. After my conversation with Biff about committing to be together for the next eighteen years, I spent my final child-free minutes on my Blackberry clearing my work calendar for the next few days. I had told my boss that we were going to take in Biff's niece and nephew for some unknown period of time and that I was hoping to count on her support through the process. She helped me think through how I should delegate projects to different coworkers so I could focus on getting the kids settled. All my colleagues stepped up and agreed to pick up my workload so I could focus on things at home. I was bowled over by their support.

WE PICKED UP Biff's mom, Kimberley, who agreed to come back to LA with us to help the kids get settled in. Lucas sat quietly in his car seat, staring out the window as we headed onto the freeway. "He seems super chill for a three-year-old,"

I whispered to Biff as I watched his face through the side-view mirror. Hailey, on the other hand, seemed to *hate* the car. She began crying right away and howled for most of the two-hour drive home.

"She's had a bad diaper rash," Kimberley said. We hadn't been able to find diaper rash cream at the kids' house, nor could we locate any books or toys to bring with us. We were hoping to create a sense of familiarity at our place with a few of their favorite items, but all I could find were a few cartoon DVDs on a bookshelf. I glanced at the kitchen and saw an open dishwasher teaming with dirty dishes, a roach running across the floor.

"This place is gross," I whispered to Biff.

"This is how poor people live, Trystan," he seethed back at me as he gathered up diapers and random socks. I felt ashamed of how I must look to him: a person of privilege who hadn't wanted for anything in his life. I made a mental note to keep working on my empathy as I tried to find another pair of shoes for Lucas, whose Thomas the Tank Engine sandals were cutting into his toes.

"Do you know where your other shoes are, buddy?" I bent over to get eye to eye with him, but he just stared at me. I began to suspect that his passive demeanor wasn't actually an indication of his "chill" nature. *Is he okay?* I wondered. I moved to pick him up, but he flinched away from me. Another mental note: *Ask before you touch, Trystan. Consent. Duh.*

"Hey, do you want a piggyback ride?" I asked. He stared at me blankly, so I got down on my knees and motioned to my back. "Come on, it's a piggyback ride, get on! Do you know what a piggyback ride is?"

He shook his head, confused, and I felt a deep wave of sadness. What three-year-old doesn't know what a piggyback ride is? Instead, I asked if I could pick him up and carry him. He nodded and I lifted him gently into my arms. I had prepared to explain to him that he was coming to stay with us for a little while, and that it was going to be super fun with lots of adventures like the zoo and the beach. But he didn't ask where we were going or how long we would be gone. He took in the commotion around him without saying a word.

WHEN WE ARRIVED at our building, I carried the kids and their few belongings through the lobby with the wrought iron railings, into the creaky elevator (which Lucas immediately hated), down the long hallway, and into our not-very-child-friendly apartment. The beautiful tall windows overlooking the secret garden were a huge safety hazard, and the sharp edges of our coffee table and bookshelves were injuries waiting to happen. Lucas's face perked up when he saw the little bed we had procured for him, but our dogs (we had three by this point) barked so loudly with excitement that he immediately started wailing in fear.

I turned to a bedraggled-looking Biff, who was carrying a sleeping Hailey with one arm while also holding a sippy cup in his hand, a diaper bag over his shoulder, a Target bag in his other hand. "What have we done?" I asked him. He was still

pissed at me for my earlier comment about his sister's apartment being gross, so he just pushed through and took Hailey
into our bedroom. I heard her wake up as he attempted to lay
her down, which meant she started crying all over again.

Trying to appease Biff, I offered to change her diaper. He
shrugged and handed me the diaper bag. I soon realized that
Kimberley had been right—Hailey had a massive infection
that smelled bad and looked worse. I cleaned her as gently as I
could and told Biff I had to take her to the walk-in clinic down
the street to get some antibiotics. He agreed to manage Lucas
and the dogs so I could deal with the diaper rash.

At the clinic, I lied and told the receptionist that my daughter was suffering from a severe diaper rash but we were visiting
from out of state and I didn't have California health insurance.
"I'll just pay out of pocket and get reimbursed later," I said
breezily. "She's in a lot of pain. How long do you think it'll be
before we can see someone?"

"This is much more than just diaper rash," the doctor said
after examining Hailey. "She has a yeast infection as well."
She wrote out a prescription for antibiotics and something else
to help with the pain. I ignored her look of judgment and got
out of there as quickly as I could.

Our living room was dark by the time we returned home
from the pharmacy, and I could just make out Lucas's sleeping
form in his new bed. A sliver of light shone out from the slightly
cracked bedroom door, which Biff had kept open in case Lucas
woke up and got scared.

I entered our room, where Biff was propped up in bed watching *The Office* on his laptop. "How did it go?" he whispered as I placed Hailey, blessedly asleep now that she finally had some relief, into the secondhand Pack 'n Play we'd been gifted. I curled up beside him and started to murmur the whole story of the lie I'd told the receptionist but passed out from exhaustion before I could finish.

I USUALLY SLEEP IN on Saturdays, but the next morning I was wide-awake before the alarm went off. I wanted to make a big breakfast for the kids, so I snuck out of bed and into the kitchen, trying to be as quiet as possible as I opened cupboards and pulled out mixing bowls. I almost jumped out of my skin when I heard a small sniffle behind me and turned to see Lucas standing in the doorway, rubbing his eyes.

"Good morning, sleepyhead," I said. "I'm making pancakes!"

I hoped for some sort of surprise or excitement, but he only stared at me warily. "Do you like pancakes?" I asked.

Nothing. I thought maybe his lack of response meant he hated pancakes, so I tried again.

"Do you want something else instead?"

I detected a faint glimmer of disappointment in his eyes, and quickly realized that (a) Lucas did indeed like pancakes, and (b) he seemed scared to get his hopes up that they might actually appear on his plate. He remained silent.

Thrilled to finally have a practical use for my years of theater and group-facilitation experience, I thought of a new system to solicit nonverbal responses from him. "How about you go like this if you want some," I said, sticking my thumb in the air. "We can do a thumbs-up for yes and a thumbs-down for no."

He lifted his arm and gave me a tentative thumbs-up. "All right! Good job!" I exclaimed. "High five!" But he only stared at my raised hand, so I gave up on that and pulled a stool up to the stove. "Here, I'll show you how I make them."

We went through the steps, and I let him help mix the batter with a wooden spoon. Biff came out of the bedroom, holding Hailey gingerly in his arms. "I put the medicine on, but it still looks bad." He brought the Pack 'n Play into the kitchen and placed Hailey inside just as Kimberley and Mark showed up to help us make it through our first full day with the kids. Lucas was watching the pancakes pop and sizzle intently when I noticed his hand creeping toward the sizzling pan.

"No!" I yelped. "Hot!"

Lucas's eyes squeezed shut and he collapsed on the ground, curling up into a ball. I dropped down to my knees beside him just as Kimberley, Mark, and Biff entered the kitchen. Biff rushed over and joined us on the floor, where I was trying to figure out what had happened.

"Lucas? Lucas? Are you okay? I don't know what happened. We were standing at the stove and he was going to burn his hand, so I told him to be careful, then he just fell down and now he won't answer. Can you hear me, buddy? Show me where it hurts?"

"He's fine," Kimberley said, sounding resigned. She stepped around the pile of us on the floor and flipped the pancakes so they wouldn't burn. "He thinks you're going to hit him because you yelled. It's best if you just hold him."

I drew him into my lap and held him as tight as I could, smoothing his hair and cooing, "It's okay, you're safe." He felt small and fragile as he made little whimpering sounds. Hailey began crying again, so I picked Lucas up and moved into the living room where it was calmer, as Biff tried to comfort her. I carried him to his bed and placed him on it. He immediately curled back into a ball, and I folded myself around him and continued my chant. *It's okay. You're safe.*

Eventually, he opened his eyes.

"Hey, buddy," I said, keeping my voice soft. "There you are."

He turned his head slightly and looked at me.

"I'm really, really sorry," I told him. "I didn't mean to raise my voice. You didn't do anything wrong at all, I was just scared that you were going to get hurt. You're not in any trouble."

I had no idea if he even understood what I was saying; I had no idea what was normal for a three-year-old, but I realized that this was not a "chill" kid at all. He was, in fact, a profoundly traumatized child who was going to need significant help from us.

"I think those pancakes might be done," I said. "Don't they smell good? Do you want some?"

All I got was his scared little stare.

"With lots of syrup?" I tried, and then held up my thumb. After a moment he halfheartedly stuck his own thumb up and climbed off the bed.

I guided him back to the kitchen, where Kimberley filled our plates. As I watched him eat, my mind raced with questions. *Isn't he supposed to be talking more? Isn't he old enough to know the difference between hot and cold? If not, what's the best way to teach him? Is he eating enough?*

And then underneath those thoughts were feelings of anger. *What kind of monster hits a child?* And beyond those questions were even darker, more disturbing feelings of hatred. *I hate them. I hate the people who did this.* I was discomfited by this deep, profound disgust. Hatred just isn't a *thing* that I do. I didn't know I was capable of it. This was dark and consuming. There was a fire beneath it that told me one day soon, I would find myself loving these children as much as anything I had ever loved before, and that alongside that love would grow a fearless protective warrior with only one job: keep them safe. I didn't know what he would be capable of, nor was I sure that I wanted to find out. But how do you parent children without also falling in love with them? And how do you fall in love with them without wanting to protect them?

As we crept into late morning, I created an Amazon wish list of everything we still needed and posted it on Facebook along with a basic outline of our situation. Biff objected to the post when he came home. "Isn't it kind of . . . I dunno . . . *needy* to ask people to send you free stuff? I guess it just feels degrading to ask for help. When I was little, we were so poor and needed so much from other people, we were taught that it was weak to actually ask for it." I assured him that I had no problem sharing our story if it meant that people might pitch in to help us, and I handled the process on my own.

That night, I settled awkwardly into Lucas's little bed next to him to read a bedtime story.

"What book do you want to read?"

When I didn't get an answer, I held up *Green Eggs and Ham* by Dr. Seuss.

"Thumbs-up?" I asked, but he gave me a thumbs-sideways.

"What does that mean? You don't care?" I asked. He nodded.

I tried reading the book to him, but he squirmed around uncomfortably, his eyes skittering around the room, anywhere but the pages.

"Don't you like bedtime stories?" I asked.

Thumbs-sideways.

"Do you ever have bedtime stories?"

Thumbs-down.

"Do you want to try again?"

Thumbs-down.

"How about I just curl up next to you for a little while, while you fall asleep?" That finally earned me a thumbs-up. I sang my favorite song, Leonard Cohen's "Hallelujah," to him until he dozed off.

Later, in bed, I finally had an actual conversation with Biff. We'd only been parenting for one day, but it felt like we hadn't spoken in weeks. There was so much I wanted to discuss with him. We had to whisper so we wouldn't wake Hailey and cuddled to keep our heads close together.

"How are you holding up?" he asked.

It was a simple question, and even though I'd been feeling proud of our efforts and relieved that more help was on the way from our friends via Amazon, I suddenly found myself overwhelmed with emotions: So, so sad for Lucas's pain and what he'd had to do to survive what was obviously a supremely messed-up situation. So angry that we had let it go on for so long before stepping in. So scared that I wouldn't be able to do this after all—that it would be too hard for me and I would cave under the pressure. I couldn't say everything I was thinking, so I just cried.

"This is really hard," I whispered. "I thought it would be fun but it's just . . . hard." Biff rubbed my back reassuringly.

"I knew it would be, but I'm sorry it's so hard. What can I do to help you feel better?"

"To help *me* feel better? It's them I'm worried about!" Without warning, my sadness turned to rage. "I'm sorry, but how did we let this go on so long? We *knew* it was fucked-up in that house. And Kimberley—she knew more than we did! Did you see her in the kitchen? They've been hitting Lucas, and she knew it was going on? This is—so fucked-up. Why didn't she—"

Biff pulled away from me.

"Why didn't she do *what*, Trystan? What could she do? Call social services? She did that. Many times. They did nothing.

Should she have kidnapped the kids? To where? Hailey's dad knows where she lives! He would just come and snatch them back! You think she didn't sit down with my sister and try to teach her what was right, how to care for them? She did. She did her best, every single day. But my sister is mentally, like, twelve years old and legally an adult, with a scary boyfriend who controls her. You have no clue what it's like to be poor, to be at the mercy of all of these systems that don't care about you. No clue at all."

Exasperated, he turned off the lights and lay down with his back facing me. This was shaping up to be the biggest fight we'd ever had as a couple. My stomach churned as I fought the conflicting urges to defend myself and prove him wrong, to appease him by apologizing and begging for forgiveness, to retreat and wait for him to come to me. Instead, I closed my eyes and took a few deep breaths, asking myself whether I wanted to be right or in a relationship. Because there is no "right" in a relationship—there is my perspective and there is his perspective, and my job is to meet him on the bridge between the two. I reassured myself that conflict is not abuse, and that even though parts of my psyche hated the turmoil, I was not in danger just because there was disagreement.

"Maybe it will all be clear tomorrow," I told myself as I fell asleep.

KIMBERLEY AND MARK went home, though we were never without support. My younger sister, Sonya, came to help us, and several friends dropped off used books and toys to keep Lucas and Hailey occupied and happy. Packages from our wish list arrived all week, including a multicolor showerhead to help Lucas with his fear of the bath and a box of diapers for Hailey. CT and Benji, who had introduced us at their brunch the year prior, showed up at dinnertime with quesadillas loaded with hidden vegetables. "To help them eat healthy," they explained as they set everything up at the table. We were profoundly grateful as we felt our community fill in the gaps in our knowledge around parenting.

Through all the messiness of friends coming over and everyone eating and reading and doing bedtimes, Biff remained the center of my universe. I couldn't stand that we weren't seeing eye to eye, so that night when everyone was finally—*finally*—in bed, I broached the subject again.

"I have thought about what you said last night," I started.

"Yes," he mused.

"And . . . I really am trying to understand all of this. My life has been really different from yours. And I'm trying to reserve my judgment while also feeling really sad for Lucas. They're both such sweet kids who deserved better. I hope you can see that my anger and frustration and sadness come from wanting them to have a good life. I'm scared about what comes next and where this all goes, and that's a good thing. I'm your partner, and I want to support you and support them. I just hope you can see that." I took a deep breath and tried to compose myself. A faint smile tickled the corners of Biff's mouth. He raised his eyebrows, inquisitively.

"Did you practice that?"

I laughed through my tears, breaking the tension. "Yes, in my head. And in the bathroom earlier. How was it?"

He reached out to hold my hand. "It was fine. And I know why you're upset. I get it. My family is messy. I've spent my whole life trying to get away from that and now, no offense, but you've tangled us all up in it again by agreeing to take these kids! It's going to be a shit show, and it's not going to get better for a really long time. I tried to tell you that in the beginning. All we can do now is ride it out." He leaned over to kiss me. I kissed him back.

"You're my favorite person," I whispered softly.

"I know." He smiled. "Now go to sleep."

IN A CRISIS, I try to create order. By the time Biff had to go back to work, I was ready to stay home with the kids. I created a schedule of meals, playtime, baths, and bedtimes and confidently taped it to the refrigerator. But I quickly learned that when it comes to caring for kids, there's only so much you can control. Every time Lucas spilled something, he would run and hide in the bathroom, which made getting out of the house nearly impossible. Hailey fought every single diaper change, to the point where it felt like I was torturing her just by trying to get her into dry undergarments!

Not that I blamed her. We received an email from Biff's aunt in Bakersfield with an attachment of a photo she'd taken of Hailey's rash several weeks earlier; she had stepped in to babysit the kids a few times and took the photo to document the problem in case it could ever be used to help the children in the future. Apparently the infection had been around for a long time. Sometimes Lucas would stand by my side and make soothing sounds to help calm Hailey down, but other times he seemed spooked by her crying and would hide in his bed. Mostly, the only way to get her to stop crying was to not put another diaper on and let her toddle around naked for a while, and by then we'd be 45 minutes past our designated lunchtime, naptime, or whatever activity I had optimistically placed on our schedule.

I didn't want to keep venting all of my negative feelings to Biff, and after a quick Google search discovered a private Facebook group specifically for aunts and uncles who were taking care of nieces and nephews. Being able to post my frustrations there helped, because many of the members understood firsthand how difficult it was to manage the anger that can arise when dealing with a partner's family and how those dynamics can ultimately affect your relationship. The online group was a much-needed outlet that I began to rely on heavily. It was a relief to know I wasn't the only one trying to process these complex emotions while also caring for children who had been neglected.

I used any spare time to research why Lucas reacted the way he did in the face of anything that he deemed threatening, no matter how innocuous it actually was. I found many articles that suggested children living in tense environments can have elevated levels of cortisol (commonly known as the "stress hormone"), which puts the brain in a perpetual state of fight or flight with no chance to settle back down to its normal resting mode. This constant heightened state can cause cognitive problems as the child grows, and I desperately hoped that we would find a way to fix whatever damage had been done to him.

WE HAD A ONE-WEEK APPOINTMENT with the social worker who had initially alerted us that the kids needed to be moved. It arrived way too fast, along with the inevitable disagreement about whether Biff and I should "de-gay" our apartment prior to inspection.

"We don't know who this woman is!" I seethed, frustrated by Biff's unwavering moral stance against taking down a particularly homoerotic photo. "Does she even know we're both men? Trystan could be a woman's name. Do we *really* want to give her a reason to take the kids away from us? It's not homophobic—it just shows bad judgment to leave this up. It makes it look like we don't know what is appropriate for children."

Biff was deeply offended by my stance. "Um, I think she is going to realize we're gay no matter what, and she probably already knows. I refuse to censor any part of my home because she might be homophobic. Lots of straight people have pictures of themselves kissing on their walls. How is this any different?"

But I held fast, and the artwork eventually came down. My older sister, Lori, who is an attorney, came down from Oregon and spent hours prepping us for this visit. Thanks to her help, we knew what to expect and were ready to put our best foot forward. Lori encouraged us to put together a binder of everything that would help make the case for the kids staying with us for a little longer. We included arrest records for everyone in the kids' old home (this ended up including convictions for spousal abuse, theft, forgery, child sexual abuse, illegal weapon sales, and drug possession). We also printed out copies of threatening texts that had been sent to Kimberley and included the photo of Hailey's infection that Biff's aunt had emailed us. As disturbed as I was by this grim scrapbook, putting it together was oddly therapeutic. Whenever I was angry about some new fact I had discovered about the kids' lives before they came to live with us, I'd find corroborating evidence of the abuse and add it to the binder.

Before the social worker arrived, we did a thorough cleaning of the apartment and dressed the kids in clothes that didn't have any noticeable stains. When I answered the door, I was instantly relieved as I realized that this social worker (who we had feared would be an older, worn-down administrator) was an engaging Black woman who I selfishly hoped would notice that we had posters up that featured some of my personal heroes: Barack Obama, Malcolm X, and Dr. Martin Luther King Jr. My hopes were dashed when Lucas marched right up to her and said, "I'm gonna kick your ass."

My jaw dropped. He'd hardly uttered a full sentence over the past seven days, and when he finally decided to speak, this is what he chose to say?! His speech was quite difficult to understand, so I stammered, "I know what that sounded like, but I think he meant to say something else."

She smiled easily and said, matter-of-factly, that she'd been to their old house on several occasions and was sure that was language he'd picked up there.

Hailey blissfully chewed on some toys in the living room while we sat on the couch and talked with the social worker. Aside from Lucas's initial threat of bodily harm, the kids behaved themselves while we did our best to reassure our visitor that they were being well taken care of. I pointed out the schedule on the refrigerator, and when Biff handed her the binder we'd created, she said it wasn't even necessary. She'd been assigned to their case for some time and was well aware of the dangers in their home.

"Unfortunately, with my county being the way it is, unless a child gets hospitalized there isn't much I can do," she explained. "I have a very full caseload and there just aren't enough homes for the kids who need them."

She took notes and asked Lucas a few direct questions about how he was doing and if he was enjoying his time with us. He gave her a thumbs-up, which earned a chuckle. We told her about Hailey's rash and how we were getting it treated.

All in all, it was a relaxed and pleasant visit, and as we wrapped up and she headed toward the door she turned back to us and said, "You two are very lucky, you know. I'm happy for you and these kids. I just got guardianship of my sister's daughter, and it took me seven years. Have a nice day."

As she left, it suddenly all made sense—why she'd broken protocol and called to warn Biff that CPS was preparing to have the kids removed. This social worker had been in our exact situation. We knew we should celebrate the fact that the meeting had gone well, but a pall of sadness came over both Biff and me. Even as a social worker she'd been unable to help her own sister, and I felt in that moment just how privileged we were to be able to step in when we did.

MORE THAN ANY of the mistakes during those first couple of weeks, one memory of a particularly rough morning stands out crystal clear: Both kids were crying and fussing, and I was short on sleep and missing my old life of concerts and movies and dinners with friends. I'd finally managed to get Hailey down for a nap and Lucas parked in front of a movie when I sank to the kitchen floor and began sobbing.

I can't do this, I thought. *It's too hard and too much. I'm going to have to tell Biff that we need to find them a different place to live.* I was so disappointed in myself and terrified about having this conversation with him. I don't remember any specific incident that triggered my decision. It was just a cumulative feeling that there was no way I could go on living the way we were, with every emotion and resource strained to the absolute limit. I thought back to my blind hope as we drove up to Bakersfield just days earlier, the swiftness with which I said, "I'm in." *I was so stupid.* I imagined telling that naive version of me-from-one-week-ago to turn around and go back to his happy, easy life where no one threw up on him, he got to sleep in whenever he wanted to, and he didn't have to invent a whole sign language to communicate with a toddler.

I was still crying quietly into my hands when I heard a small sound and looked up to find Lucas standing in front of me. I was mortified at the idea of him seeing me show any sign of weakness—I'd been raised in a home where parents never shared that level of emotion with their children—and tried unsuccessfully to wipe evidence of my tears away.

Since I was on the floor and he was standing, we were eye to eye, and he reached his hand out and touched my cheek. "It's okay," he said. "It's okay. It's okay."

I realized that all of my time spent reassuring him that he was safe with me—it had all been worth it. As he repeated my own words back to me, my sadness turned to joy. I reached my arms out to him and he collapsed into me. We held each other there on the kitchen floor, me crying and him probably very confused about what was going on. I put my feelings of shame at showing weakness aside and absorbed the moment for what it really was—two people expressing love and empathy for each other. I knew that if Lucas was capable of this at such a young age, we had a pretty good chance of ending up okay, no matter how difficult the road ahead might turn out to be.

Notes from Life in Our Family

Get Flexible.

Is there a more critical word when it comes to parenting? I learned in the early days that each kid needs something different, and trying to force my expectations of normalcy onto them would surely backfire. Hailey needed time to heal from her diaper rash and needed to be held *all the time.* Meanwhile, Lucas simply could not handle anticipation. It would overwhelm him so much that he would obsess over what was coming up. Biff and I eventually stopped talking to him about plans, period.

When it came to Lucas, we used a crucial bit of advice from our friend Vesta Van Patton-Dunn: to learn to accept and live with who he *is*, rather than who I think he should be. It's a lesson I'll likely be working on forever.

With every fight you have with your children, ask yourself, "Is this worth it? Can I change my own approach and not deal with this fight every time?" Sometimes it *will* be worth it, and you can choose the battle. But most of the time, you can make an adjustment and not have to deal with that particular struggle ever again.

Get Resourceful.

It's not your partner's job to support you when you're in a rough spot if the issue you're dealing with is a tense one for both of you. Whenever you feel stuck, ask yourself, "Am I utilizing all of my resources?" Remember that the internet and social media can be resources. Your family and friends may be great resources. If your partner is on their own journey, go on one of your own and seek the support that you need elsewhere. It's okay to lean on your partner, but it's not their job to be your only source of support.

Get a Reality Check.

Remember that if you have a partner, you likely chose them because you trust them and their judgment. I definitely should have taken Biff more seriously when he indicated how incredibly stressful the weeks we brought Hailey and Lucas home were likely to be. If I had lowered my expectations for myself and truly buckled down in preparation for a period of crisis and chaos in our lives, that period would have undoubtedly been easier. If your partner is giving you signs that you need to adjust your expectations . . . then maybe you should rein them in.

Get Humble.

I confess. Even though I work very hard on this, it's hard for me to stay as nonjudgmental as I would like to. I still find myself wondering why Biff's family made the choices they did. My mind was quick to come up with accusations about this family and their lifestyle because I was terrified that Biff didn't realize how dysfunctional it all was. I was terrified that slowly the dysfunction of his family would poison ours. Judging them was my way of distancing myself from them and the mess I saw. It was my way of making myself feel better while I tried to protect myself and this shaky informal sort-of-family I was suddenly in charge of.

Unsurprisingly, none of that helped. In fact, my obsession with finding fault in Biff's family made it even harder to be a good parent to Lucas and Hailey, and a good partner to Biff. I spent so much time trying to convince Biff that his family was a wreck, when I should have been focusing on how I could be helpful. We all would have been much better served if I had found a way to do what Biff had done—accept that not everyone behaves the way you want, and some things are never going to change. Yes, there is dysfunction and even abuse, which Biff was absolutely aware of, but the answer is to show up and help.

We got into a toxic pattern, with me bitching and moaning about how terrible his family was, which only set him up to defend them, and that would frustrate me to no end. We would go round and round at odds with each other, rather than being on the same side.

Your partner's family is their family, and as long as your partner is committed to breaking the unhealthy patterns in their family of origin . . . let your judgment go. It won't serve anyone.

Get Information.

There's so much to learn about the ways that trauma impacts the brain's development. We hadn't really mastered the art of parenting traumatized kids yet (does anyone ever?!), but we *did* learn that working to avoid their triggers—the events that had caused negative associations in their minds—was the best way to get through the days while seeking resources for them to heal.

If you're parenting kids in nonideal circumstances, you may have to learn while doing (or do while learning). Don't be afraid to ask for help. I had my therapist friends on speed dial during this period, was reading voraciously, and had already started to make calls to preschool programs that might be equipped to handle special circumstances.

Get Self-Aware.

Figure out what *your* individual triggers are. What situations are likely to cause you to not be able to think straight? One of my triggers is feeling as though I don't have a lot of power. When I find myself facing these kinds of scenarios, I work to find awareness—to not get trapped in the situation, but instead to notice that I'm in it and to try to do something useful to distract myself. When dealing with our looming legal fight, a situation with so many aspects I had no control over, I found something I did have control over and could take action on—the binder. Collecting text messages from the involved parties, researching arrest records—those were all things I could do, and that process created the illusion that I had any power at all in this completely overwhelming situation. When you find yourself stuck, ask yourself, "Is there something I can *do* to take control here? Is there a way I can surrender and accept that I don't have control over many things in my life? How can I be helpful and create or do something useful?"

CHAPTER THREE

HOW WE DO MARRIAGE

—

We were at a concert when I figured out how I would propose to Biff.

We had crappy orchestra seats in the old Downtown LA theater where folk legend Ani DiFranco was performing. We'd been caring for Hailey and Lucas for several months and were in desperate need of a night away, so we planned a "staycation," with relatives watching the kids overnight so we could have a nice dinner, see a show, and stay at a hotel. It had been a beautiful evening together, and as the first chords of a sweet love song began, I looked over at Biff's face, gently illuminated by the reflection of stage lights, and thought, *Wouldn't it be cool if Ani pulled us up on stage so I could propose to him?* I wondered if I could make it happen. I surreptitiously pulled up Twitter on my phone to see if I could send a DM to Ani DiFranco or her team, but their security settings prevented me from connecting with her directly. I put the phone away to enjoy the rest of the show, but the seed of a proposal continued to grow quietly in the back of my mind.

AFTER SEVERAL YEARS together, I was officially in my thirties and Biff was in his "early late-twenties." Our more responsible friends had begun to think seriously about marriage and family, and for some reason they were coming to *us* to ask for proposal ideas. My friend Jaan came into town from DC and over dinner at our house solicited our advice about his proposal to his girlfriend, Priyanka. Biff was quick to respond.

"You'll want to do something really dramatic," he suggested. "A thousand roses in her apartment." I was dismayed by this extravagant idea. A *thousand* roses? Was this his idea of an appropriate proposal?!

The following week, my friend Maceo met up with us for drinks and let it slip that he, too, was planning to propose to his girlfriend.

"What do you think I should do?" he asked us. Again, Biff jumped right in.

"How do you feel about a hot-air balloon?" he suggested. My heart sank. If I couldn't get ahold of Ani DiFranco's people, how could I ever come up with anything close to what Biff was suggesting to our friends? *Maybe it's better to wait until we get everything settled with the kids. A time when there's no drama.* But as time ticked by and we encountered more interviews with social workers, additional court dates, and legally mandated waiting periods, it started to seem like maybe a time with no drama was never going to come. In fact, I thought, maybe a wedding would be a good distraction while there's so much legal maneuvering going on. It would be something positive and fun for us to focus on, instead of wrangling our family. So I decided to do it; I was going to propose. It was clear that I couldn't get Ani DiFranco on board, but I did have someone famous and glamorous to ask—Our Lady J.

I had seen Our Lady J perform in New York in 2007 and quickly became a die-hard fan. A young trans woman who had trained as a concert pianist, J wrote songs about enacting revenge against transphobic men and told stories about being raised in an Evangelical household in the south where her parents found and confiscated her Bowie and Prince records, lining them up on a brick wall and shooting them with a shotgun. She was the kind of person who could bring a room to silence just by entering it, inspiring whispers of "Who's that?" Unapologetically commanding, elegant, and fearless—she was everything I dreamed of being.

When Biff and I had just started dating, J moved to LA, and I sent her an email asking if she wanted to be involved in a project I was working on (this was 2011).

Much to my surprise, she wrote back right away saying she would love to plan something with me and asked if I wanted to get coffee sometime. Turns out the move to LA had been a hard one; she had been a celebrity in New York's cabaret underground (the same community that produced Lady Gaga) and it was jarring to move to a new city where no one knew who she was. "I don't have any friends here," she confessed to me over brunch, as other patrons gawked at her six-foot-tall presence. "I had no idea it would be so lonely." We were fast friends, bonding over our shared devotion to trans elders and our belief in the power of music and story. Our friendship extended past the project I invited her to partner on, so when I approached her a year later, asking if she'd be willing to help me propose to Biff . . . she was thrilled to help me make a plan.

I DIDN'T KNOW if he would say yes. We had joked about getting married, and during the initial months of parenting Hailey and Lucas we had secured a domestic partnership in order to communicate to the judge how serious we were about our relationship and how stable our household was. But as we signed the documents, we had decided in no uncertain terms that the domestic partnership was a pure formality and *not* a marriage or a wedding. We knew that when we *did* get married, we wanted it to be something we could share with Hailey and Lucas: a formal event, rather than the uncere-monious process of signing forms in a bleak mail center on Hollywood and Vine (which is what the domestic partnership was). It was not unlike the time when Biff bought me a ring for Christmas and prefaced the gift by saying it was *not* an engagement ring.

"It's not that I don't want to get engaged," he explained. "It's just that if I ever propose, it won't be as simple as giving you a $30 ring in a box at Christmas."

Okay, I thought. *Then how* are *you going to propose to me?*

Whenever I suggested that *I* might be the one to propose, Biff snorted and huffed. "Oh, you think because you're the more masculine one that you're automatically supposed to propose to *me*?" I was totally bewildered. Did he want me to propose to him, or would he be offended if I did? *Was* I being sexist by wanting to propose? What did marriage and a wedding really mean, anyway? Occasionally he would show skepticism and abject hatred of the concept: "Why would anyone need the government to sign off on their relationship? What is a wedding other than a really expensive, wasteful party, anyway?" But I had the sense that a proposal, a wedding, and marriage were all things Biff had been taught not to expect from this world, and that his distaste for them came from a protective instinct he'd learned over the years. *If you won't give it to me, that's okay because I didn't want it to begin with.*

Of course we said "I love you" to each other, and of course we couldn't imagine a life apart. After all, I had already committed to spending the next eighteen years with him! But the idea that there might be "the one" who completes you just seemed intellectually, numerically, scientifically stupid. Biff had seen the women in his family do so many ridiculous things because they believed in the idea of love and commitment beyond all sane judgment; his mother had stayed with his abusive birth father for years, even after the man was arrested for embezzling from the police department where he worked, even after they had to flee their town out of embarrassment and shame, even after he became addicted to cough syrup and threatened her and their children on drunken, belligerent nights. She believed in her love for him and believed it was her duty to stay. And after Biff's dad left, his mom married a man (her second husband, before marrying Mark) who was so unaccepting of Biff's queerness that Biff had to leave his hometown altogether when he was still a teenager.

Biff could give or take love, and he could give or take marriage, and he could give or take "forever." He had learned that forever was a lie, and that you should always be prepared to see the signs of dysfunction and flee.

"I don't want to need you," he would sometimes say when we were feeling particularly close and connected. "I don't want to need anyone or anything."

What is marriage but an agreement that you need each other—that your lives are intertwined and that you are both better for it? Would Biff see marriage as a trap, another snare that would make leaving me more difficult?

It had been months since we signed the domestic partnership papers, and we'd been parenting Hailey and Lucas that whole time. We still didn't know what the future for us as a family was, but I wanted to convince him that it would be okay to need someone else, and that sometimes, people do stick around. I wanted to show him, by proposing, that his life could be different from his parents'. But would he believe me? I couldn't be sure until I asked him. So I asked him.

IT WAS THE SUMMER of 2012, and Our Lady J had a concert at Casita del Campo, a Mexican restaurant and performance venue in Silver Lake, on the east side of LA proper. I had emailed, called, and texted all our friends to let them know about the proposal. At my request, Biff's parents even came down so Kimberley could be there when it happened (Mark agreed to watch Hailey and Lucas for the evening). In my pocket I could feel the heavy weight of the titanium ring I had custom made for the occasion; the jeweler agreed to let me purchase it on a payment plan, and I'd been sending checks every month for half a year. We parked the car and held hands as we walked into the venue.

As we sat down, Biff noticed how many of our friends were in the audience with us.

"Dang, I guess everyone we know loves Our Lady J!" he exclaimed. "Is that Samir? I didn't know he was into her!"

"Yeah, I guess so," I agreed, trying to sound casual.

CT and Benji were there. So was my boss who had watched our relationship blossom from the very beginning, as were half a dozen of Biff's friends from the social group he ran. The lights went down, and the show started. Our Lady J emerged into the spotlight on the tiny stage and began her usual schtick: funny, touching stories about her life and childhood, along with Dolly Parton covers and original songs with sweeping piano refrains.

Her feet pounded the pedals as I began to sweat. Then she said the phrase I had been waiting for.

"Ah, love. I love love. Do we have any lovers in the audience? Is anyone here in love?" A smattering of hands went up. She shaded her eyes to look out at the crowd, pretending to notice me for the first time. "Is that . . . is that Trystan out there? Are you two in love? Come on up here, you guys!"

This was it. Exactly as planned. I grabbed Biff's hand, and we made our way down the aisle and up onto the stage. J handed me the microphone, and I took a deep breath. A confused hush fell over the audience as our friends awaited the question and strangers tried to figure out what was happening.

"Biff . . . as you know, I love you very much. And I never want to be without you. I've loved getting to know you and having so many adventures with you. And I promise you, if you say yes—" I fumbled around in my pocket and pulled out the ring. "I will give you a whole lifetime of adventures." Shaking and sweating, I awkwardly got down on one knee and held the ring up. A collective gasp shook the room as everyone suddenly understood what was happening.

"Will you marry me?"

Biff's face registered complete shock as he took the ring and stared blankly at it. The spotlight made it hard to see him fully and I was still holding the microphone in my hand, but I knew he hadn't answered either way yet. Time slowed to a crawl.

What if he says no? In front of all these people? What was I thinking? Why couldn't I just let a good thing be? Why did I have to complicate everything? I finally shrugged my shoulders, trying to silently say to him, *Well? Is that a yes?*

He shook his head slightly as if to wake himself out of a trance and exclaimed, "Yes. Of course! Yes! Of course!" I stood up to kiss him as the audience exploded into cheers. J began to play her next song, and I returned the mic to its stand. Biff pulled me back to our seats, his face glowing in a way I had not seen before, and he kept looking at the ring I'd given him as if he could not believe it was real. We settled back in our seats, my stomach humming with excitement.

"Did you really not know? Was it a real surprise?" I asked him quietly.

"I had no idea! Is that why all our friends are here?" he whispered, as J wailed away in the background.

"Yes," I told him. "Your mom, too. I've been working on it for months."

He smiled and squeezed my hand.

"I love you," he said.

"I love you," I replied.

And we began to plan our wedding.

GAY MARRIAGE WASN'T LEGAL in California at the time, nor was it legal in Oregon (where we were about to move), so the legal part of getting married wasn't even on our radar. It was really just the ceremony and party we were interested in. We wanted a celebration with our friends and family, a time to stop and recognize that we had found each other and cobbled together a family in a world where such things shouldn't really be possible. We wanted a wedding, and I wanted a formal ceremony, a ritual to signify our commitment.

Biff, however, was not on board with anything traditional at all. "No, we're not doing a ceremony. Walking down the aisle? Writing vows? Why would we do that? Let's just have a party! A reception with food and cake and dancing and really good cake!" But I was determined to have a *wedding* wedding, and Hailey and Lucas were excited as well. I felt there must be a reason that every culture engaged in some kind of ceremony to consecrate the union of two people (or more, depending on which culture you're talking about). There must be something sacred, a magic of sorts, that happens when people gather and engage in ritual to honor a relationship. And I wanted that. Even if it was seen as emulating straight culture, even if it was rooted in sexist notions of women as property, even if it reeked of oppressive monogamous ideals. I wanted it, and the kids wanted it, and we begged and pleaded for months until Biff finally caved.

"Okay, fine. But let's not just do what everyone always does. Let's think about which traditions actually work for us and which don't, and we will cut the stupid ones." That was okay by me, but we would need help. I was on the phone with my mom when she suggested it.

"Oh, you know who could officiate? Annie McManus. She would be great!" I knew right away that my mom was right. Annie was like a pixie come to life—light and airy and full of joy. She was a leader and facilitator at an intergenerational summer camp we went to every year on Orcas Island, off the coast of Seattle. Biff and I adored Annie; hell, *everyone* adored Annie. She led a weekly multifaith gathering in Olympia, where she lived, so we knew she had a firm grasp of many traditions and would be superb at holding conflicting truths at once. She was also a hospice nurse, which meant she was adept at managing gut-wrenching decisions with grace and ease. We had known her for several years and had seen her juggle complex family dynamics at camp, and she'd been our most trusted parenting coach during particularly difficult times with Lucas.

She would encourage: "When he gets upset, just bear witness to it. Don't feel obligated to fix it for him or change your decision—just be with him and be present to his pain without affirming or prolonging it." Annie's words of wisdom never felt accusatory or shame inducing. She would always reassure us that we were doing a great job with Lucas, no matter how much it felt like we were failing. I believed she would be an amazing officiant, and Biff agreed.

She said yes right away, and we set aside time to talk through the ceremony with her. I came prepared with meaningful objects from our relationship, hoping to paint a picture of our love so she could help build a ceremony that truly represented what we were to each other. These included Post-it Notes I had hidden all over the house before leaving for a conference, a calendar Biff had made for me with photos and quotes from

Hailey and Lucas on each page, and a box of notecards Biff had filled with things he loved about me. We also talked through the many challenges our wedding would present; we each had family members who didn't get along with each other and we needed her help navigating those treacherous waters. Finally, she asked us to share what we hoped the wedding would feel like to us, what it meant to us, and what we wanted to look back and feel great about. We left the meeting feeling excited and inspired for the wedding and what it could mean for us and our community of support.

It felt good to be asking friends and family to come participate in something fun instead of dealing with our latest crisis.

ON THE DAY of the wedding, a clear blue early-summer day even though there had been rain in the forecast, we awoke at my parents' house in Victoria, British Columbia. We had driven all around town the day before, buying the flowers, picking up the cake, and confirming the delivery of mics and amps. After months of planning, our wedding day had finally arrived, and I fought to stay calm as tempers flared and deep-seated family resentments came crashing down all around us. *I can't control what they do*, I reminded myself of Annie's words. *I can only control what I do, and I will act with integrity.* Before I knew it, my brother-in-law was playing a delicate refrain on his guitar and it was time.

The wedding party started in the living room, while the guests sat in rows of chairs in the backyard meadow waiting for the ceremony to begin. To my delight, Biff had decreed that we could, in fact, walk down the aisle; as the music swelled, he and his mother linked arms and began the procession toward Annie, who stood where the dais would be if we were in a church. Hailey blew bubbles as she walked with my friend Heather, and Lucas held the rings as he walked with Colleen, Biff's dear friend (who is also my foster sister). I linked arms with my mom and, when it was time, she and I walked down the aisle to join the rest of the wedding party in front of our guests. Biff and I had eventually agreed that being "given away" by our mothers was an important symbol of leaving one family cluster and truly committing to another. We decided that our moms should do the escorting, since we were both close to our mothers and his birth dad wasn't in our lives at all. I remember feeling outside of my body as my mother guided me forward, beaming with pride and excitement and, I later learned, relief.

"Now I can stop worrying about you," she told me during the reception as we ate chocolate cake. "I can truly let you go and trust that you'll be okay." I wanted to tell her that I was a grown-ass man in my thirties whom she didn't need to worry about in the first place, and that I had been with Biff for years and that a wedding wasn't a magic wand that would change our relationship. But I stopped myself, realizing that in some ways, a wedding *is* a magic wand that had changed our relationship. Maybe it wouldn't change the way we felt about each other, but it would change the way the world viewed us as a couple. And it was a magic wand for my mom, someone not at all rooted in biblical tradition. Somehow, the symbolic act of giving me away lifted a burden off her shoulders as she released the primary job of carer and protector of me, handing that responsibility over to Biff.

She did feel light and joyful on my arm as we walked down the aisle, and we parted ways as I took my place next to Biff. Annie said a few words, none of which I remember but all of which were, I'm sure, perfect. We had invited both of our "best men" (Heather and Colleen) to speak, and Kimberley, too. Their words are lost to time, the whole ceremony overwhelmed by what happened next. It was my mother's turn to take the stage, and I had no idea what she was planning to say.

Every time I had tried to ask about her portion of the ceremony, she was uncharacteristically evasive. "I have a plan," she assured me. "Don't worry." There had been too many other details to fret over, so I hadn't pushed it or thought about it much. Biff noticed it, too, but encouraged me to trust her. I couldn't help but wonder what she would say. Would she read from the book of Ruth? We aren't religious, but in *Jane of Lantern Hill*, there is a sweet passage that invokes Ruth's promise of *Whither thou goest, I will go; whither thou lodgest, I will lodge; thy people shall be my people*. I always thought it was beautiful, and it had a special meaning in my family. Or maybe something from Rumi? My mother had never shared her spiritual beliefs with me, but I suspected the ancient poet might resonate with her worldview. I held my breath as she stepped forward.

But she did not use the mic when it was handed to her. She set it down on a chair and nodded to our guests, all of whom stood up. She nodded to my brother-in-law, Justin, who was still seated with his guitar in hand, plugged into the speaker system. He began to play a refrain that was very familiar to me: the first chords of Leonard Cohen's "Hallelujah." I looked at Biff, bewildered.

"What's happening?" I asked him out of the side of my mouth.

"I don't know," he whispered back with a shrug.

Then our guests all took out sheets of paper and began to sing in unison.

> *I've heard there was a sacred vow*
> *That lovers make, as you do now*
> *But you don't really need this promise, do you?*
> *It goes like this*
> *Through ill, or health*
> *The pain of loss, the joy of wealth*
> *Together you are singing Hallelujah*
> *Hallelujah, Hallelujah,*
> *Hallelujah, Hallelujah.*

As is true for many in North America who were born in the 1980s, I feel a close personal connection with the song "Hallelujah." I sang it to Lucas at bedtime every night since the first night he came to stay with us and used it to soothe him during times of distress. But as I listened to this wedding version, I realized that these weren't Leonard Cohen's lyrics. So, whose were they?

Your faith was strong, you needed proof
You saw Biff acting quite aloof
His beauty in his T-shirt overthrew you
You sat yourself beside his chair
Attracted by his long pink hair
And from your lips he drew that Hallelujah
Hallelujah, Hallelujah,
Hallelujah, Hallelujah.

Holy shit, I thought. *It's my story. It's OUR story.*

Though, dear, you brought me lots of fun
Sometimes it's hard to raise a son
And watching you with Lucas, I see through ya'
You think it's hard when they are small
That isn't anything at all
The teen years cause a frenzied Hallelujah
Hallelujah, Hallelujah,
Hallelujah Hallelujah.

I couldn't believe what was happening. My restrained, profoundly unsentimental mother had taken my favorite song and rewritten the lyrics to tell the story of raising me, watching me fall in love, and then witnessing me raise children of my own. She called me her "son" in the song, and though I was well into my thirties and fully secure in my transgender identity, the word rang out above the others. *She sees me as her son.* But the song wasn't over; the guests—our friends and family—kept singing.

Climbing was your favorite thing
Trees and ladders, anything
You never let the breathless falls get to ya'
And, Biff, I'm glad he fell for you
He dreamed of kids, you brought him two
They call him Dad and I cry, Hallelujah
Hallelujah, Hallelujah,
Hallelujah Hallelujah.

It's not that I thought my mother was heartless. I didn't. I had witnessed her selflessness in hundreds of ways big and small throughout my childhood, into my adolescence, and well into adulthood. She had tolerated years of teenage backtalk and sass, had pummeled us with lessons on politeness, determination, and discipline. She had welcomed Hailey and Lucas into her life as her grandchildren without a thought about genetics. When we struggled to make ends meet over the years, she sent us money. When Biff's brother needed methadone, she donated to the crowdfunding campaign. But throughout all of those moments of support, she never once showed real tenderness or vulnerability. It just wasn't her way. She never cried or used flowery language. My dad's voice always catches whenever he and my mom say goodbye to us at the end of a visit, and as he tries to hug us and tell us how proud he is of us for all we've done, my mother drags him away before he can "make a fool of himself." "Come on, Clay! Traffic!" she says, clearly uncomfortable with even his subtle display of emotion.

Biff, I ask you take his hand
Be good to him but understand
He used to feel alone before he knew ya'
I've seen him give this love a chance
For Love can be a victory dance
It's a warm and it's a joyous Hallelujah.
Hallelujah, Hallelujah,
Hallelujah, Hallelujah.

Her heart had been there all along, showing itself in her actions—the acts of service large and small that all added up to a lifetime of boundless, unconditional love I hadn't really seen until that moment. While I was waiting to find Biff, certain he didn't exist at all, my mother was watching, waiting with me. While I longed for a partner and children, my mother was there, longing with me. While I was falling for Biff and learning to love all of who he was and let him love me and all of who I am—she was witnessing it all. And she had put it all into this, her grand gesture of love: the best wedding gift I could have ever received.

We'll do our best to help this last
Support your love as time goes past
We'll tell the truth, we didn't come to fool you
Married life needs work we know
But through the years your love can grow
With nothing on your tongue but Hallelujah
Hallelujah, Hallelujah,
Hallelujah, Hallelujah.

Though marriage is a pathless trek
Sometimes you soar, sometimes you wreck
You cannot let the petty things get to ya'
Now, Biff, I'm sharing him with you
To trust, to hold, to see him through
I hope you'll both keep singing Hallelujah
Hallelujah, Hallelujah,
Hallelujah, Hallelujah.

As the song wrapped up and I wiped the tears from my face, I turned to see Biff and his niece and nephew, who were now our son and daughter. I saw his mother and, out in the chairs, his stepfather. And their grandchild, Emilee, whom they were raising. The realization hit me hard—Biff was trusting me with *all* of this. His whole life. His care and well-being, and that of the most precious things in his life: Hailey and Lucas. His love for me was so all consuming that he was willing to put his faith in me—to trust, to hold, to see him through—after an entire lifetime of fierce independence and emotional solitude.

What could I ever do to be worthy of this love?

OUR VOWS, TOO, are lost to time and a messy attic. I know he promised to be faithful to me, a nod to my old and bitter fear that he couldn't possibly stay with me-and-only-me forever. I know I said the words "I choose you," a reference to our first shared TV show obsession, *Six Feet Under*. I know we read vows to Hailey and Lucas, and did a "one, two, three, whee!" with each of them, a ritual we knew they would understand as fun, if not sacred. And I know that as Annie pronounced us married, we kissed and I took Biff's hand and raised it up in a victorious salute as we walked back down the aisle, a married couple at last. But the details are fuzzy. What is most prominent in my memory is the humbling, terrifying, exhilarating feeling of being deeply, profoundly loved, and the promise I made to myself that I would do everything in my power to be worthy of it.

Notes from Life in Our Family

Get Creative.

If there is one thing queer people know, it's how to get creative. The systems weren't built for us—marriage, tax forms, fertility clinics. So we've had to DIY the crap out of everyday systems. But deciding to do things your own way isn't just for queers anymore. Anyone can, and should, take a critical look at cultural norms and institutions to decide which they want to be a part of and which aren't suiting their way of life. Ask yourself: Are you participating in systems the way *you* want to, or the way you've always been told you're supposed to?

Why shouldn't women propose to men? Why shouldn't people be friends with their exes? Why do dads still walk their daughters down the aisle? Why do non-Christians get married in churches? Why must weddings cost so much money?

There may be perfectly legitimate reasons for these things, but in all seriousness . . . if you want to do things differently, don't get sucked into tradition or hurting your mom's feelings. Just pretend you're queer (if you aren't already) and imagine that you have the opportunity to do things however you want, on your own terms, without any rule book. Which parts of your life would you want to stay the same? Which would you change?

CHAPTER FOUR

HOW WE DO ADOPTION

—

"Permanent guardianship isn't really permanent," I said to Biff. "We need to adopt them."

A year after our wedding, we packed up and moved from Portland to New York City, chasing a job offer I couldn't turn down. The salary was nearly double what I had been making at the Task Force, and I had felt it was time to move on from there, anyway. The new job as director of development at Immigration Equality was high paying and high stakes—I had to raise millions of dollars or LGBTQ clients were deported, with fatal consequences. I thought I could handle the pressure. It turns out I couldn't. I didn't have what I needed to succeed and was in way over my head. Perhaps because I felt so much insecurity around my new job, I began to worry that something might happen to separate us from the kids.

"But why?" Biff asked. "What do you think might happen if we don't adopt them? My sister doesn't have the resources to file the paperwork and go to court to take them away. She'll never be able to do that. She couldn't even make it to that final hearing." I knew, in a sense, that he was right; it was unlikely that she would be able to successfully regain guardianship. But my older sister, Lori, kept pressing me on it. She was a family lawyer and had seen all kinds of shocking and heartbreaking separations over the years.

"She's a pretty girl," Lori warned. "All it would take is for her to convince one guy with half a brain cell that she's been screwed over by the courts, and if they can look stable for a few months and you get a homophobic judge . . . no amount of great parenting can save you and you could lose the kids. It seems impossible now, but I've seen way worse."

There's a reason lawyers are stereotyped as all doom and gloom. They see people at their lowest points and are trained to look out for the worst-case scenario. Lori really got into my head, and I persisted in pressuring Biff. Finally, he relented and allowed me to email our LA lawyer, Elise, to ask her how much it would cost to file for and secure a full legal adoption of Hailey and Lucas. Elise didn't mince words: "All told, even with my reduced hourly rate, we're talking $10,000 minimum. Let me know how you'd like me to proceed."

I was gutted. I wasn't sure how we could possibly come up with $10,000. Biff and I sat at the table in our Brooklyn apartment and looked at our family budget. Even though

I was making more money than I ever had before, we had Brooklyn rent, weekly groceries, subway fare, credit card debt, and homeschooling supplies for the kids. There just wasn't anywhere we could cut back. My salary, which had seemed astronomical when I accepted the job, was barely covering our basic expenses. The rent, even in the modest neighborhood of Bed-Stuy, was more expensive than any apartment we had ever lived in. But we also couldn't imagine living even farther out in Brooklyn where rent was more affordable, as it would have made my daily commute to the financial district even longer and would have taken Biff even farther away from necessary parenting and household requirements like parks and grocery stores. As it was, Biff had to take the subway anytime we needed groceries, and it was nearly impossible to carry back enough for a whole week with two kids in tow. Occasionally, he would splurge and take a cab home from the shopping trip, but how do you get a stroller into a cab? Not to mention a car seat for Hailey, who was still a toddler!

My inability to perform well at work slowly eroded all self-confidence I had built up over my years of organizing at the Task Force. On most days I was the first person in the office each morning and the last one to leave each night, but I still wasn't able to please my new boss. Every day there was something new I had messed up, and no amount of overworking could solve it. Everything was hard in New York, and we were barely scraping by emotionally and financially. Biff tried to think of ways he could bring in money, but we couldn't come up with anything he could do while also parenting two young children full-time while I worked 70 hours a week.

We were stuck.

IT ALL CAME TO A HEAD one night after I had spent the afternoon in a detention center with a colleague, observing a legal intake with a lesbian woman from Africa whose mother had forced her to undergo female genital mutilation after finding her with another girl. She was fourteen when that happened and had spent the subsequent two years meandering across the globe, trying to make it to America. She surrendered herself at the border and was promptly placed in an immigration detention center where cases were so backlogged that she'd been languishing for six months in what was essentially a prison, awaiting a hearing. As we left the detention center after the meeting, my colleague told me that this woman didn't stand a chance of securing asylum because she didn't have any proof that she was actually gay. "She doesn't have any photos of herself with any girlfriends, no love letters, nothing." *Only, how could she? It was forbidden!* I was immensely frustrated at a system intent on further punishing those who had already suffered so much.

I arrived home in a daze, overwhelmed by grief and powerlessness. Picking at my microwaved dinner, having missed bedtime with the kids, I asked Biff about our adoption prospects. We'd had the conversation before, but I couldn't help bringing it up again.

"Could we put it on a credit card and pay it off over time?" I wondered.

"We maxed out our cards moving here and are already paying as much as we can every month on those. I think we're just paying down the interest at this point." He sighed. "It's just not the right time. Maybe things will get easier in a few months or years and we can do it then." He patted my hand and headed off to bed. "It's late."

I stayed at the table, looking at our budget and bank statements. *Okay,* I thought. *So, we can't bring in more money and we can't spend less. What other resources do we have?* I was determined not to let money stand in the way of giving Hailey and Lucas the security they deserved. The more I thought about the impact their adoption would have on them, the easier the solution seemed to be. *Our community!* I remembered. *We have our community!* I pulled up my computer and began drafting a fundraising page.

"Love (and Money!) Makes a Family." I stayed up for hours that night, typing up our story in the text box of a GoFundMe page. I pored over Facebook photos of us together, chose the best ones, and uploaded them. I may have been failing as a development director, but I did know how to ask for money. I had learned at the Task Force that all you need to do is tell your story honestly, in a way that others can relate to, and then get them excited about what the future can hold. Let them know how they can help that future become a reality, and that's your whole job right there! Whether it's securing votes or donations, the formula is the same. I proofread the page once, then I hit publish.

It was after 2:00 AM when I crawled into bed next to Biff. I fantasized about a day when I didn't cry in the bathroom at work, when I was home before the kids were asleep, when I had the time and energy to be a better partner. I felt drained of joy, bereft of hope, and I couldn't stop thinking about the dark, distant eyes of the young woman in the orange jumpsuit I had sat with earlier that day. *Is this what my life is now? Powerful enough to know how much suffering there is in the world but powerless to stop it?*

But when I woke up the next morning and opened my laptop, a tiny glimmer of happiness returned.

"You did what?!" Biff exploded at me. He was furious that I had set up a fundraising page without checking with him first.

"I set up a fundraising page, but guess what—we raised all the money we need for the adoption." I tried to get the words out fast, hopeful that it would soften the blow. Biff *hates* asking for help or having someone ask for help on his behalf. Hates it. But I had taken a chance, hoping that it would pay off—and it had.

"It . . . it did? Who donated? How much money did we raise?" Aha! I knew it would be worth the risk.

"I set the goal low, for five thousand dollars. And we already hit it. People are asking us what the full amount for the adoption will be, and I'm going to tell them it's ten thousand dollars. We may be able to do it, after all!"

Biff began to protest, claiming that fundraising for something personal is like begging, and that people who aren't truly destitute shouldn't be asking for the resources of others. But when I showed him the comments sent in by contributors, he softened.

"Look—'Thank you for letting us be a part of your family's story.' And another one—'I have been waiting for you guys to tell me what I could do to help!' People want to help," I reassured him. "It's empowering to them. I tried to tell you—" But I could already see his anger fading away. He took a deep breath and then sighed.

"Okay," he said. "Okay."

WE HAD SOME UNEXPECTED HELP in ultimately reaching our fundraising goal. My job in New York City ended abruptly, and we hurried back to the West Coast, relieved to be heading home but also a tad bruised by our New York experience. I quickly secured a new job at a youth-serving organization in Portland and ended up taking the bus to and from work each day. This gave me time to dig back into podcasts, which I hadn't been listening to much. I fell in love with so many new storytellers! The position at the top of my playlist was quickly awarded to Hillary Frank, host of *The Longest Shortest Time*. The podcast was ostensibly about parenting, but she found a way to make each episode completely enthralling, touching on issues of guilt and shame, relationships, racism, and so much more. I loved listening to her interviews and stories, never once imagining how profoundly Hillary and her podcast would impact our lives.

One evening, as I pulled the cord to notify the bus driver that we were approaching my stop, the producer for *The Longest Shortest Time* hopped onto the show to remind listeners that they were always looking for new story ideas, especially about nontraditional parenting experiences. *We have a nontraditional parenting experience*, I thought, as she provided instructions on submitting a story idea. As I walked home, I pulled up the story submission webpage on my phone and dictated our story into the text field. I covered the basics: We were two men who had taken in our niece and nephew and were now parents kind of by accident, which is rare for a gay couple. I hit submit just as I got home, and I quickly forgot about my attempt to secure a spot as an interviewee on my favorite podcast.

A few days later, an email from a producer on the show landed in my inbox. They were interested in our story and wanted to hear more. We scheduled a call, and I excitedly told her more about our weird parenting journey. As I was explaining our story, she cut me off.

"Actually, Trystan, I'm going to ask you to stop. I'm totally sure I want you to be on the show, and I don't want you to overtell the story. Would you be available next week to record an interview?"

I couldn't believe it. I was so excited. Given what I knew about their listeners, I had a hunch that our story would play well. Hopefully, I thought, a few hundred people would hear about our family and it would inspire them to support LGBTQ families or adopt a child or to otherwise gain a deeper understanding of people like us. This was my chance to do some real good in the world. I had never heard a story like ours, so I was optimistic that it would be interesting to others. I never imagined it would help us complete the adoption.

That first episode about our family, which Hillary called "The Accidental Gay Parents" (a nod to a discussion in which we mused about how rare it was that a gay couple become parents "accidentally"), was released in June 2015. Much to my delight, listeners demanded to hear Biff's side of our story, so he was interviewed for part two, which was released a month later. Some fans of the show found our fundraiser online, and we hit our $10,000 goal.

We were going to be a forever family after all.

WITH THE MOVE to New York and back, the flurry of fundraising for the adoption, and becoming B-list podcast celebrities, Hailey and Lucas continued to be the center of our world. Lucas was in a day program part-time and was homeschooled by Biff the rest of the week. He would have been in kindergarten, age-wise, but wasn't yet meeting the benchmarks for kindergarten readiness, so we decided to wait a year, continue to educate him at home (in addition to his half day of in-person class), and put him in kindergarten when he was ready. He still struggled with transitions, disappointment, and dysregulation, so we wanted to keep him home as long as possible. He also started exhibiting obsessive behaviors. He would choose a word or phrase, like "property" or "missing," and root around in the idea for months at a time.

He would ask, "This my property?" Only he couldn't pro-
nounce the word correctly, so he sounded like he had a thick
Boston accent. "Why this your prah-puttyy?" "Who prah-putty
this be?" He didn't seem to be able to unlearn something
once he'd convinced himself that was the right way to say it.
"We go to hims house?" "I no have ice cream?" If he learned
the words to a song incorrectly, it would take months and
sometimes years for him to understand that those were not
the right words. It was hard to know when to gently correct
him, when to passively model the correct language, and when
to just let it go.

As we all settled back into Portland, Biff and I struggled
to reconcile our relationship as co-parents. After all, I'd been
unavailable as a true partner for many months. This was when
we discovered the art of discussion over email. I had wanted
to know more about his homeschooling methods, like what he
did during the day, what the kids were working on, whether
he was including letters and numbers or if they were playing
and going on adventures as methods of teaching. I didn't have
strong feelings about any of these approaches, but I wanted to
be able to participate and weigh in as their other parent. But
even the most germane of questions was greeted with defensive-
ness. "Why are you asking? Do you think they're not learning
when they're with me? They're learning! We do things!" Biff
would say. No matter how gently I tried to inquire, I was met
with resistance. So, one day I tried a new tactic.

I spent a long time composing a thoughtful email to him, outlining my respect for him as a parent and my admiration for his ability to stay home with the kids. I made it clear that I thought he was doing an amazing job and that I understood that at this age, academics shouldn't be a focus for Hailey and Lucas.

"But I want to be really clear: I am also their parent and I have a right to be engaged in their life and their learning. I should be able to ask you how things are going without being snapped at, and if I'm not asking in a way that feels good to you, just tell me how to change and I'll change," I wrote. "I don't like this cold war that's happening, where I'm not allowed to even ask what you guys are up to. I promise I won't judge you, but I want the chance to weigh in whenever and however feels appropriate to you. I want to support you, and it's difficult right now because of the way you're responding to me."

I read and reread the email to make sure I wasn't making any vast generalizations (Biff hates it when I say anything that begins with "you always" or "you never"), and to make sure that I was focusing on specific actions and their impacts on me.

1. What you did that I don't like

2. Why I don't like it

3. What I want to be different

I used that basic formula, made sure that it was written as delicately as possible, and sent it off to him. I didn't receive an email response, but that evening after the kids went to bed he sat down and talked with me. He acknowledged that he had been defensive because he was insecure about his parenting. He wasn't sure he was doing a good job and wasn't clear about my role in the situation. Was I his boss? Were the kids his boss? Was he our boss?

When we first moved to Portland with the kids, Biff decided not to get another social work job; he wanted to be a full-time parent so the kids would have as much support as possible. Even though we'd been to New York and back he'd stayed in this role of full-time parent, and he still wasn't sure that he was doing it well. But he promised that he would try to be more open to my input. I promised I wouldn't try to boss him around, not that he would have let me get away with it, but I said it anyway.

"Let's start now: What did you guys do today?" I asked.

He shared about their time at the museum and told me how he was working on letters and colors with Hailey, and numbers with Lucas. "I'm most interested in social skills with Lucas, so I'm going to take him to a play group on Thursday to see how he does with other kids."

We continued talking openly into the evening. It was the first of many, many, *many* conversations about how to give the kids what they needed, and the beginning of an already treacherous journey as we tried to navigate our differing approaches to Lucas's unique challenges. I learned then that I had to be delicate when bringing feedback to Biff; the protective mechanisms he had built throughout his life now extended to his role as a parent, and even the most gently worded inquiry could feel like an attack. Sending emails became our own way to work through our differences; it was a vital survival tactic for us to communicate.

BEFORE WE KNEW IT, we had started the legal process of adoption. This meant that we were back in the orbit of Biff's sister and her boyfriend, back in the world of lawyers and judges and investigators, back in strategy-and-planning mode. At this point, we'd had custody of Lucas and Hailey for four years, but the adoption process brought back memories of how difficult the first year had been—constant court dates and lawyer's meetings and investigations. It had come to a pause once we were awarded permanent guardianship, but now we were heading back into battle without ever really healing from the first one.

Everything in the child and family court system is designed to keep children with birth parents, to reunite children with birth parents, and to protect birth parents from losing their parental rights. We quickly learned that in order to proceed with the adoption process, we would have to submit letters from friends, teachers, bosses, and doctors. When I asked my primary care provider to submit a letter stating that I was in good health, she did so gladly—and included a paragraph about her observations of me as a parent. Lucas was super into bodies that year, so I would sometimes bring him with me to medical appointments. He loved looking at the equipment and watching me get shots or tests. My doctor shared that I had been an engaged, attentive parent to Lucas, and added that she strongly supported our petition for legal adoption.

While it was frustrating to jump through all of the hoops in the legal system, I tempered my frustration by remembering why those rules were in place. Many atrocious things have happened in America with regard to parents and children. Even though the process was exhausting, I tried to remind myself that these obstacles existed for a reason and we were just collateral damage.

AFTER MONTHS OF FILLING OUT FORMS, at long last we had a court date to finalize the adoption. The kids' birth mom had broken up with her longtime boyfriend and moved to Utah to be with a man she'd met on Facebook. He ended up being abusive, so she was staying at an emergency shelter somewhere in town. While in Utah, she decided to voluntarily terminate her parental rights. It took dozens of crackly pay phone conversations. She would call us and say she would sign the forms, and then she would disappear for weeks with no trace. Then, out of nowhere, Biff's birth dad came into the picture and decided he would "save" his daughter. He sent her some money so she could come and live with him for awhile, and she got herself a phone. Before she left Utah, Biff coordinated with her and a local adoption attorney to sign the papers. She missed the first two appointments but finally showed up at the office. They called us to let us know it was done. When we received the bill, the attorney had reduced her fee by half out of recognition of the importance of adoption. We were grateful.

Meanwhile, our LA lawyer was attempting to serve Hailey's biological dad with parental termination papers (he wasn't Lucas's birth father), but he was in the wind. None of the addresses we had for him were current . . . and then the system pinged—he showed up in jail, which meant he could be served papers. Since he was in jail, he had all the time in the world to object to our request for adoption. He was given a free, court-appointed attorney who conveyed a series of convoluted requests on his behalf. He agreed to terminate his parental rights under the condition that we allow him to write to Hailey, would send him regular photos and updates on her life, and provided him visitation.

We were incensed. These demands were particularly egregious given that he hadn't seen her for three full years by that time (nor had he ever requested a conversation or visit with her before), and the discussion tied us up for several weeks as we tried to decide whether to give him any concessions. If we said no outright, our lawyer told us, he could deny the parental termination altogether and we would have to engage in a legal battle to convince the courts to terminate his rights unwillingly. But if we gave him anything he had asked for, it would mean opening the door to having him in our lives forever. We reluctantly decided to allow him to send letters if he would like, to be shared with Hailey at a time and place of our choosing. (As of this writing, six years after this allowance was made, he has yet to send her a single letter.)

Dealing with Biff's sister's transience and her ex-boyfriend's manipulative requests took a lot out of me. Biff and I fell into an old pattern: I was exasperated, and he was neither shocked nor surprised by the behavior of his relatives. I wanted so desperately for him to hate them, but he refused. He was steadfast in his acceptance of their messiness, resigned in the knowledge that they would not change—so why waste energy wishing things were different?

THE NIGHT BEFORE our adoption hearing, we flew down to LA and stayed with friends for the night before trekking out to the children's courthouse east of the city. It was a muggy July morning, and a handful of friends met us outside. I was completely convinced that something would happen to ruin the day, but Hailey and Lucas were excited and bounced around the lobby in their fancy dress-up clothes; Lucas's front teeth had just fallen out, so his tongue poked through when he smiled.

Our names were finally called, and we traipsed into the courtroom: Biff and I, Hailey and Lucas, our lawyer, CT and Benji, and my best friend, Heather. The judge looked over her glasses at us and said, "Well, what do we have here?"

Too young to understand courtroom decorum, five-year-old Hailey declared, "It's our love family!"

Taken aback and clearly quite touched by this bold statement, the judge cleared her throat and began the ceremony.

Hailey and Lucas were each given an "adoption bear" by the court, and they hugged them tight to their chests as the judge asked Biff and me to solemnly swear to love and care for them as if they were born to us. We both said, "I do," she offered to take a photo with us, and then . . . it was done.

We burst out of the courthouse like skittering balls of electricity, laughing and crying and hugging each other. Our friends congratulated us, and our lawyer wiped away tears. I was overcome with emotions—relief and joy and also sadness. I would never again be young, footloose and fancy-free. I would always be responsible for these amazing humans, and I wasn't sure I deserved that trust. *What if I let them down?* I thought. *What if I can't do it?* And I held their mother in my heart, too, angry though I was at her. I wondered if she knew that today was the day she said goodbye to her children.

On the steps of the courthouse, I held Hailey and Lucas tight in my arms.

"Do you guys know what this means?" I asked them. They nodded.

"Yes," Lucas said proudly. "This means we're a forever family."

EVERY YEAR, ON SEPTEMBER 4, we celebrate Chaplow Family Day to honor the day when the kids first came to live with us in 2011. I created the ritual to show Hailey and Lucas that it will always be okay for them to talk about the story of how they came to be our children. Every year we retell them how it happened, and every year they ask new questions. "Was I cute when I was little?" "Tell me again—why couldn't my mom take care of me?" "Was she sad when we left?" So many questions, not all of them with easy answers. But I never promise them easy answers. Just a commitment to be with them in the questions.

Notes from Life in Our Family

Get Talking.

Whatever your story is, you have a chance to make an impact with it. Even if you don't *think* you have a story . . . you do. Imagine what would have been helpful for you to hear when you were younger. Imagine what you *did* hear that inspired you to think or act in a new way! Know who your audience is and learn about their perspectives and values. Whether you want to talk about your lesbian sister or transgender son, or you'd like to share your journey around racism or antiracism, or if you're a survivor of trauma . . . don't keep your story inside!

I never could have imagined the impact our story would have on the world and am so grateful that I chose to share my story way back when. I had lots of training in storytelling and messaging, but that's not necessary. Don't be afraid to give it a shot—you can make a difference in someone's life by opening yourself up to them.

Get Motivated.

According to one of my heroes, the rapper Stic.man—an avid follower of the *I Ching*—improper motivation is rooted in ego and greed; it asks, "What can I get out of this?" It also drives decisions made out of fear and desperation. Projects rooted in improper motivation are likely to fail or even backfire, says the *I Ching* (as told by Stic). Proper motivation, on the other hand, is rooted in service and connection to others; it asks, "What can the world get out of this?" It drives decisions made to empower and strengthen others and is much more likely to be successful.

Whenever I'm scared or stuck or can't see a way through, if I reorient my thoughts away from myself and my limitations, and instead focus on the positive impact I can have on those around me as a result of my actions, an entire universe of possibility opens up before me.

Until I had really thought about what adoption would mean for Hailey and Lucas (a safer, more secure life) instead of what it would mean for me and Biff (less fear), I couldn't see what the path forward could be. Whenever you're at a critical decision point, or get stuck or feel afraid, examine your motivation. Is it proper or improper? Can you focus on the outcome of your actions, rather than what your actions will mean for you?

Get Honest About Adoption.

As an adoptive parent, so many aspects of raising children are complicated. It's hard to reconcile the joy of parenthood with the knowledge that your gain is someone else's loss. You're a parent only because someone else lost their child. If the child was taken away from a birth parent, somewhere along the line, the parent failed that kid, those systems failed that family . . . so many breakdowns have to happen.

I was petty toward our kids' biological mother. I know I was. I held her responsible for their abuse and neglect. I still do. No matter how many times Biff and I face her poverty and drugs and intergenerational abuse—I cannot forgive her for what she allowed to be done to her children. They, and I, live with the impacts of her decisions every single day, and we will for the rest of our lives.

I also recognize that I was petty because I was insecure about my role as their parent, and I must be honest with myself about that. I don't like it when they ask about her, because I fear that on some level, they wish she were still their mother. I fear that I will never be enough of a parent for them. When they ask about her, of course I do everything I can to be neutral and to not show my personal feelings. I answer their questions to the best of my ability, given their age and what I think they can understand. And then I reassure myself that my worst fears are definitely true: they *do* wish she was still their mother, and they will always wish they weren't taken away from her. Every child wants to be loved and cared for by their first parents. The grief of losing that will always be with them, and it's not their job as kids to assuage my grown-up fears. It's their job to go on their grief journey, just as it is my job to walk alongside them. I have gone on my own grief journey without them ever knowing.

None of that progress can happen unless you're honest with yourself about your complicated feelings and can center what is best for your child rather than what feels good to you. It's hard, hard stuff. But hey—no one ever said parenting would be easy.

CHAPTER FIVE

HOW WE DO CONFLICT

~

As we were in the final stages of the adoption process, I again felt the pull of a baby. I found myself reaching out to other trans friends who had given birth to ask about their experiences. I began rigorously searching for academic research on trans fertility and even emailed my dad (who is an endocrinologist) asking for his opinion on the safety of trans pregnancy. He sent me six articles on the topic, one of which clearly showed that trans pregnancy is safe and advisable; I would simply need to stop taking my hormones well ahead of getting pregnant and ensure that I had strong social supports in place. Online, I found a group focused on transgender men and pregnancy and eventually worked up the courage to write my first post, asking for basic information, like how long I should be off testosterone before trying to get pregnant. Everyone was warm and welcoming, happy to answer my questions.

Once I had assured myself that trans pregnancy was, in fact, perfectly safe and medically advisable, I turned my attention to Biff. Though we'd been together many years, I had never told him about the baby dreams I'd had early on in our relationship. He had always made it clear that he couldn't understand why anyone would choose to bring new children into the world when there are so many others already out there that need love and a safe home. Besides, with Hailey now five and Lucas at eight, Biff and I were getting our first taste of independence. It no longer felt like we had to spend every waking moment just trying to keep them alive. They could play in their rooms alone and give us a little space to breathe, read, and nap—all the tiny luxuries that we'd once taken for granted but had sacrificed to give them a home. I thought about bringing up the conversation but just couldn't find the right time. When *is* the right time to bring a brand-new idea to your partner, especially when you're pretty sure the answer will be no?

THE "RIGHT TIME" presented itself in Spring 2015. The non-profit I was working for owned a sprawling, classic Oregon summer camp where they often held gatherings. I was invited to a work event there, which was basically a free weekend family vacation in exchange for a little physical labor. I was the first on staff to sign up.

When we arrived on-site, Biff and I were assigned trail maintenance duty. Hailey did crafts with a counselor, and Lucas went hiking with a couple of the older children and a guide. Biff and I gathered downed branches from the paths and chopped them up for kindling. The forest floor was soft and wet, moss clung to the trees and hung down into the path, and far away we could hear the excited laughter of kids playing in the meadow. We worked quietly alongside each other, happy to be outdoors and getting exercise in the fresh air.

I may not have been talking, but there was much I wanted to say. Many parents have fantasies about what they'll do with the extra space in their home once a kid is old enough to move out, but Biff and I had always said that once Lucas left, we wouldn't want to turn the spare bedroom into a home office or workout space. We'd want to keep it as a bedroom not only for when Lucas returned home to visit, but also as an available space for foster kids in need. I hadn't planned to bring up having a baby to Biff but being out in that calm forest, it felt like the right time to broach the subject, and I used the spare bedroom as my way in.

"Hey, so you know Lucas's room? What would you think," I said cautiously, "about maybe when he moves out, keeping that room available for a baby?"

Biff now claims that he immediately felt both sides—a little bit excited and also concerned about everything that would entail, but as I remember it, he didn't express either of those in the moment. Instead, his response was, "What?!?"

I began to dial it back fast, attempting to make my idea sound as though it were a passing whim inspired by some friends' recent experiences. "Oh, well, it's just something I've sort of been thinking about. I know it probably seems out of nowhere for you, but it's just something I've sort of been tossing around, you know, as maybe a possibility for us. Way down the road."

"I mean, I guess it is," he said, but I heard the doubt in his voice. "And I'm sorry to jump the gun. I love you very much, and if this is something you really want, then of course I will consider it. But my first instinct is no. That sounds like a terrible idea."

His tone implied that sure, we could talk about it, but it wasn't actually going to happen. I was heartbroken, having spent months gathering information about pregnancy, talking to my father, and otherwise making up my mind about having a baby. I hadn't realized that he would feel blindsided by this proposal, having never imagined the possibility of a biological child in all his years of picturing his own future. And meanwhile, I had built up this fantasy that involved me asking him about a baby and him falling to his knees and enveloping me in his arms, exclaiming that yes, he would love to make a baby with me and had thought I would never ask.

As Biff often says, I'm a dreamer . . . and he's a realist.

"Yeah, just something to maybe keep on the back burner," I stammered. "I know we've got enough going on already."

"I *will* think about it." We fell silent and resumed clearing the hiking path for the hundreds of children who would walk through it that summer.

WE WENT BACK AND FORTH on the baby topic over the coming months until, on the advice of a friend, we put a moratorium on the subject and agreed to each think it over independently. We were at an impasse, both so certain that our opinion was the right one that conversations were beginning to feel more like arguments. We drifted toward summer, silent on the topic of a baby, and tried to focus on work and spending quality time with Lucas and prepping Hailey for first grade.

We may not have been *talking* about a baby, but it was definitely on our minds. Biff has always had to be stubborn and self-driven in order to survive in his family—with so few adults paying attention to him—and the world, which wasn't designed with the needs of a small effeminate boy in mind. I have often found it hard to break through that shell. As time dragged on and no decision about a baby was made, I was plagued by the thought that our marriage would always consist of us doing things however *he* wanted them, with my needs on the back burner. The baby question only reinforced my fear that I would never be truly valued and seen as an equal in our partnership. I felt myself growing distant from this person I so deeply loved.

As he considered this question of a baby, Biff was silently working through every single concern you can imagine and more. He later explained that most straight men go through life knowing that one of the paths they might end up on could involve getting a woman pregnant and having a child, whether they wanted to or not. Heterosexual guys prepare their whole lives for how they'd feel if that happens, if only on a subconscious level. Biff had never in a million years imagined that he'd have a partner he could have a baby with. Even as he came to know my trans friends who'd given birth, it still seemed like something *we* would never do, so it just . . . didn't come up in our conversations. And it didn't come up in his mind.

IN AUGUST, WE TOOK THE KIDS with us to Beloved Festival, a four-day camping event featuring sacred music from around the world, living art installations, and extravagant workshops and performances (like aerial yoga and ecstatic dance). I knew it would be a total hippie fest straight out of *Portlandia*, but it was the only kid-friendly festival I could find, and I was looking forward to it.

On day two, Biff went off on his own to take a yoga class while I took the kids on a walk through the festival grounds. We arrived back at the tent at the same time, and Biff pulled me inside while the kids made stick drawings in the dirt nearby.

"Okay," Biff told me. I was confused.

"Okay what?" I asked.

"Okay, we can have a baby," was his response.

I was stunned.

"What? What changed your mind?"

"Eh, I don't really want to go into it. I just did. We can have a baby if you want to."

And that was it. Though it wasn't the way I had imagined it would be . . . we were going to have a baby.

I CALLED A TRANS FRIEND whose partner had given birth recently, looking for recommendations on fertility clinics. He said they'd had a good experience at the Providence Maternal Care Clinic. I knew that most trans guys would bristle at the name ("maternal" is quite the gendered word, after all) but figured I couldn't be picky, or I might end up with no medical support at all. I called them to make sure they took my insurance and went in for a pre-pregnancy checkup. When I walked in, the woman at the front desk asked if I would prefer to wait in their private waiting area in back; I didn't mind the awkwardness of being a man in an office full of women, but it was nice of them to offer. Already we were off to a good start. When it was my turn, they checked my vitals and gave me an ultrasound to make sure everything looked okay in there. The OB-GYN was kind and respectful. At the end of our appointment, she shared that I would be their first trans pregnancy and asked if I could recommend a facilitator they could hire to train them on trans inclusion so they would be prepared to support me. I was thrilled to be asked (and doubly thrilled that she hadn't expected me to do it for free, which is a common request). She looked at my test results and gave me the green light to start doing what

I needed to do! I eagerly wrote down the advice she gave me: start eating healthy, exercise, don't skimp on sleep, take prenatal vitamins, and stop taking testosterone.

I'd done enough research by then to know that stopping testosterone was an important and necessary step, and I wasn't worried about what might happen when I stopped. I'd been taking it for over ten years by then, and my body had undergone enough changes that I didn't expect my beard to start falling out or my voice to change its timbre. Those transition effects (facial hair and voice change) are largely permanent once they happen (which is why it's harder for transgender women to remove their body hair and change their voices if they wish to—once testosterone has hit the body, either during puberty or as part of a transition process, many of its effects are impossible to reverse). So those crucial elements of my gender expression would stay put, though a menstrual cycle and rapid mood swings were about to begin.

There's much more information about reproduction available now for people who are transitioning than there was when I started out. In fact, it's supposed to be standard practice for doctors to make sure that anyone transitioning under medical care fully understands the impact on fertility, particularly since transitions are increasingly happening at a younger age due to increased acceptance and wider understanding. Unfortunately, I still hear from trans people all the time that their providers are giving them incomplete or wholly inaccurate information about their fertility.

Prior to any kind of hormone therapy or gender affirming surgery, doctors *should* discuss fertility and refer their patient to a specialized center that can preserve sperm or eggs. Although testosterone usually prevents ovulation when taken properly, there is strong evidence to suggest that taking testosterone has no effect on the quality or quantity of eggs. If someone on testosterone wants to get pregnant—or gets pregnant unexpectedly and plans to carry the pregnancy to term—then they should stop taking testosterone, as doctors have reason to believe that it can be bad for a developing fetus.

I thought I was prepared to deal with the biggest effect of stopping testosterone: the return of a menstrual cycle. What I wasn't expecting was the brutal roller coaster of emotions that ensued.

For trans-masculine people like me, going on testosterone is often referred to as puberty and menopause . . . at the same time. All the hormones that would have kicked in during adolescence, had I been male-assigned, are suddenly playing catch-up. It's basically ages 12 to 16, all smushed into six months. And most of the estrogen-based hormones simultaneously cease production, so it's also ages 55 to 65, smushed into that same six months. I had some vague memories of this process from when I first started testosterone at age 20 and assumed the reverse process (stopping testosterone) would be just as difficult. *But I'm older now,* I thought, *and I've been through enough therapy that I'm pretty sure I know how to handle my emotions.* I was prepared to steadily name my feelings for what they really were, use calming breaths, and get through it while the testosterone worked its way out of my body and the estrogen process kicked back in again. Easy peasy.

Turns out I was completely unprepared. When Lucas bounced a basketball against our house it was like a cannonball being shot from right next to my head, over and over again. It was infuriating. Biff crunching popcorn next to me in bed, Hailey whining about an injury we weren't sure was real—the slightest little thing could suddenly make me so frustrated that I'd have to go walk around the block so I wouldn't have an outburst. The worst part was a sudden inability to communicate what I was feeling, particularly to Biff. Looking back, I know it must have been exhausting to have a partner who couldn't handle any amount of frustration, emotional overwhelm, or discomfort. Biff did his best to be patient with me and to explain to the kids why I was so on edge, but it could not have been easy. I tried to apologize as much as possible, in large part to assuage my own guilt: I felt like an unfair burden on everyone. Was having a baby a stupid, selfish idea? My mother had encouraged me to consider why I was making this decision and putting so much at risk—a happy relationship, a beautiful family. I began to doubt that this was the right thing to do, after all.

The doctor I spoke to at the Maternal Care Clinic told me that it might take a couple of months for my menstrual cycle to kick back in (three to six months on average), but with all the emotions I was feeling I figured it would show up at any moment. A month went by, and nothing. Then another, and another, and still nothing. I started to worry and wondered if I'd been on testosterone for so long that it might never come back. The data simply doesn't support this fear, but there is still so much we don't know about trans bodies, and it turns out that anxiety can creep up whether or not reassuring evidence exists.

I soon discovered that my body was fine. There was just some extremely basic seventh-grade biology I'd completely forgotten about. I had believed that I wouldn't be able to get pregnant until after I got my first period. But one of the handy pop-quiz tricks to remember how the reproductive cycle works is to think of a menstrual period like the period at the end of this sentence. It marks the *end* of the cycle, and unbeknownst to me, my body had released a fertile egg sometime in October and it had done its thing with one of Biff's swimmers.

I only started to suspect that I might be pregnant when I suddenly began to put on weight. I hadn't undergone top surgery, and I noticed that my chest was swelling and tender to the touch. I went to the drugstore, picked up a test, peed on the stick, and got the plus sign.

I kept waiting for the wave of excitement but felt . . . nothing.

Similar to the moment when I'd told Biff that I'd wanted to have a baby with him, and then again when he finally agreed, I expected fireworks of happiness that simply never came. But this time, it was I who felt strangely unemotional, not Biff. Then the panic set in.

WE WERE *SO* not prepared. Biff and I had both been looking forward to a gradual process with lots of time to plan and organize. Not only did I assume I couldn't get pregnant until after my first period, but I thought it would take several more months after that for anything to happen as my body continued to adjust hormonally. Yes, Biff had agreed to have a baby with me, but it was still very much an ongoing conversation, and my mood swings of late hadn't exactly fostered a lot of productive discussion. A small, scared part of me worried he might even be angry.

I couldn't sit with this information alone, though, so I texted Biff and made up some excuse as to why the kids and I wanted to stop by his work. When I arrived, I went into his work bathroom with a new pregnancy test I had picked up on the way and peed on that stick. I came out of the bathroom and asked him to meet me outside, where I showed him the plus sign. The shocked look on his face matched everything I felt inside. Biff describes it as suddenly seeing a giant clock ticking; we only had a limited number of months to prepare and figure out how we were actually going to do this.

Maybe it was my need to snap us out of our terrified state, but I said, "Let's tell the kids!"

"Are you crazy?" he said. "We don't know what this is going to look like. Anything could happen. My mom said you're not supposed to tell anyone until after the first trimester."

"Fine. Well . . . yay? Right?"

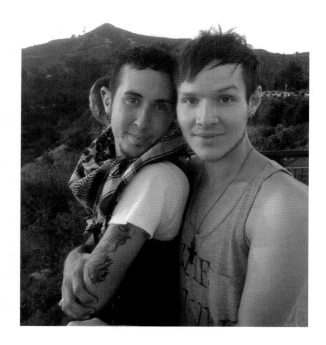

The first photo taken of me and Biff, at Griffith Park in LA, in 2009

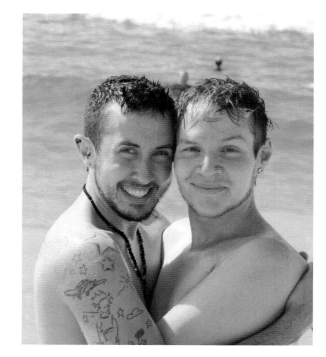

Our last photo before Hailey and Lucas came to live with us, on the island of Kauai, in 2010

Top: The first photo we took together: me, Biff, Hailey, and Lucas at the LA Zoo, in 2010

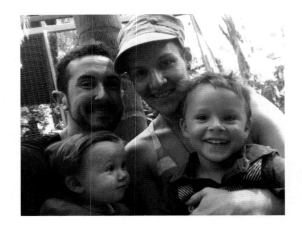

Bottom: Us with Hailey at our wedding, in 2013

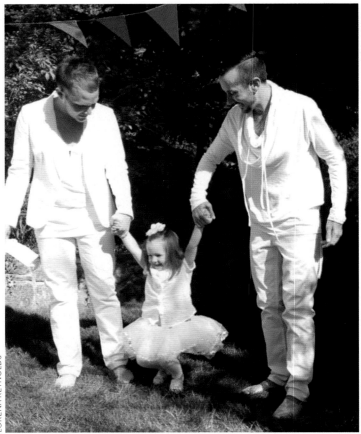

LORENA REYNOLDS

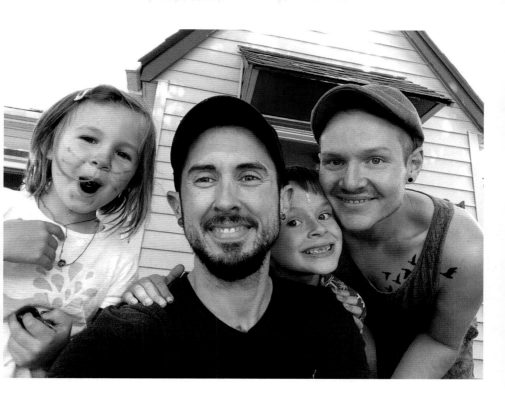

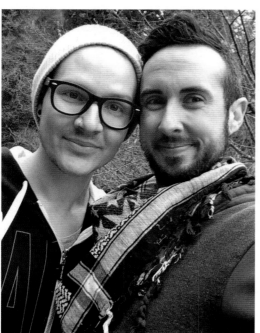

Left: Me and Biff by the Sandy
River at Camp Namanu, when
I tentatively asked if we could
have a baby, in 2015

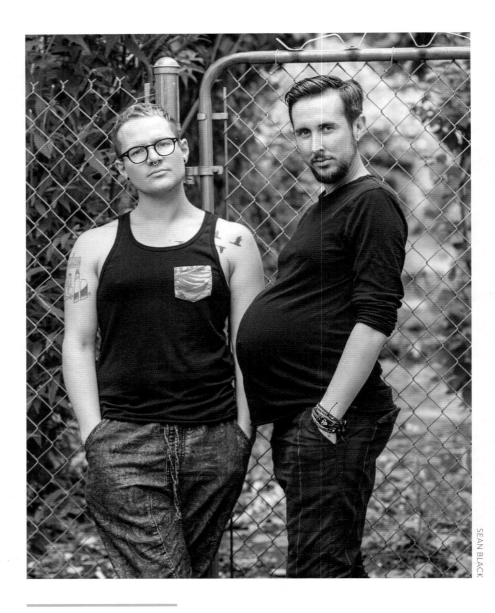

A very pregnant me, with Biff
in our backyard, in June 2017

Right: Me with my father, Clay, in the hospital before Leo was born

Below left: Our first photo with Leo, including me, Biff, and my father

Below right: My mother, Janet, with Leo, in 2017

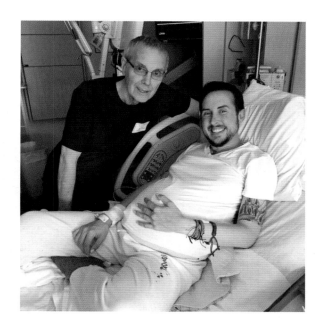

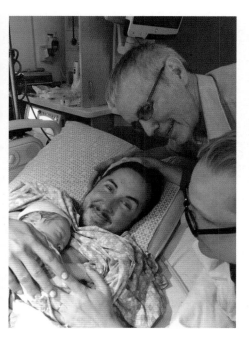

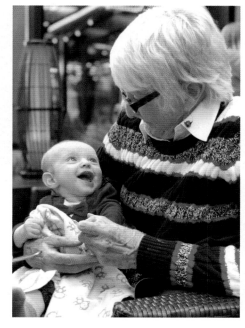

Me on stage delivering my
story for The Moth Mainstage
in Brooklyn in 2018

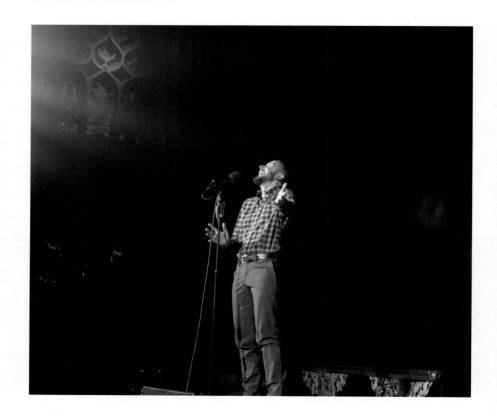

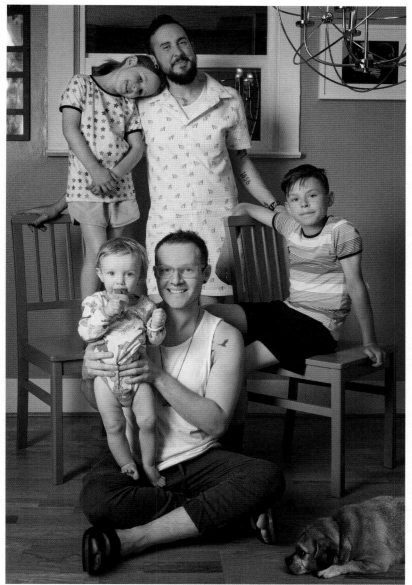

All five of us: Hailey, me, Lucas, Biff, and Leo—
plus our dog, Marley—in our home, in 2018

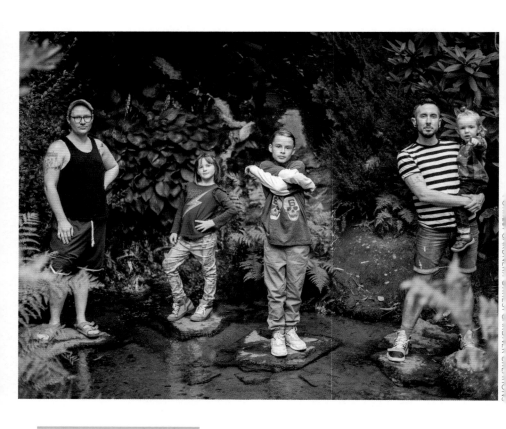

All of us in Portland: Biff, Hailey,
Lucas, me, and Leo, in 2019

"Yeah, of course. I mean, I guess this means it was meant to be. There's no question now: We are supposed to have a baby." He sounded exactly as flat as I felt.

I WENT BACK to the clinic for a blood test to confirm that I was definitely pregnant. My hormone levels suggested I was about four weeks along, but the doctor told me to schedule a follow-up appointment in two weeks for an ultrasound to make sure. Without the start of a period to go by it was a harder to gauge when exactly this had happened.

One thing was for sure—I'd been knocked up long enough for pregnancy hormones to start kicking in, and I was also still experiencing mood swings from going off of testosterone. It became harder and harder to keep my cool about anything that pissed me off even the tiniest bit. When Hailey requested a third hug in a ten-minute span of time or Lucas launched into one of his hours-long pouting jags, I would blow up at everyone with a "I can't live like this anymore!!!" before storming out of the house for a drive. I knew that my emotional ups and downs were becoming hell for Biff, and I felt terrible but couldn't seem to keep it under control. And then there was my sense of smell.

I've always been incredibly responsive to scent. I'm that annoying person in your office with the aromatherapy machine churning out all kinds of herbal fragrances. Within a few days of discovering I was pregnant, I discovered, much to my chagrin, that I could smell everything. And I mean *everything*. Once

I was riding the train on my way to work and could tell that the man four rows over hadn't brushed his teeth after a breakfast of black coffee and Cheerios with almond milk. Walking past any garbage can on the curb was a full-on stink bomb assault, and there were times when I'd enter a restaurant and then turn right around and leave, scared I might vomit due to the smell of some perfectly normal menu item that my nose believed was toxic.

Not all food smelled gross, thank god, because my hunger cravings were equally out of control. As Biff would yawn and say he was going to bed, I'd say, "Cool, I'm going to go make a bunch of toast. Want some?"

Sometimes I'd find myself wide awake at 2:00 AM making a beeline for the refrigerator, and throughout the day I devoured three times my usual amount of food. I craved McDonald's french fries all the time. This was not normal. I'd never liked them before, and our family never eats there, but I'd order two large fries, dump a packet of salt all over them, and then toss the empty bag in the neighbor's trash so no one would find out.

Aside from the fries, my hunger ended up being one of the few places where Biff and I found common ground—he's a snacky person in general, so he was more than happy to stay up late with me to make midnight nachos. Biff describes this period as his favorite out of the whole pregnancy process, and he definitely put on a few sympathy pounds (which we were both okay with).

Even when we were getting along, we were still unable to truly talk about the pregnancy. We'd cover lots of other ground, but that was the one area where we mostly kept our worries to ourselves. The few times we did try to engage, it never ended well. For example, I still really wanted to tell the kids. I hoped that getting them excited would finally make me and Biff excited and we could turn the pregnancy into something we could all be joyful about, but he continued to shoot it down, telling me that it was a terrible idea.

His concern wasn't just that it was still way too early; he also pointed out that we were asking them to suspend a lot of typical notions about what's normal when it came to us having a baby. "They're already going out into the world every single day a little bit different because their family doesn't look like other families, and I'm not ready to ask them to take this on too," he said.

On a rational level I knew what he meant, but pregnant-and-no-testosterone Trystan did not see it that way at all. I took everything he said as hurtful, as though he didn't believe in us strongly enough to handle having a baby. "Fine, I guess we'll just do it your way then," I huffed. "As always." And stormed out of the room. Not my finest moment.

For some reason I was still holding on to all my romanticized notions of pregnancy, all that weird stuff like expecting him to wait on me hand and foot, put his ear on my belly and sing songs to my womb. He wasn't giving me any of the emotional support I desperately craved, but his late-night nacho construction skills helped smooth things out a little.

I confessed all of this to him later, once we were back on track. He gave me a weird look and said, "Since when have I ever sung to you? I've never done that. That's not who I am."

It turns out he *was* excited about the pregnancy in his own way, but he was also in his own head about how the pregnancy messed with his identity. Not in any of the ways one might expect though. The easy diagnosis is to think, *Oh, the gay guy is freaked out because now his husband is pregnant.* It had nothing to do with that, and everything to do with the role he'd carved out for himself in the family we'd already made.

Over the course of our relationship, I had never stopped working full-time, and had in fact begun to do consulting work on top of my full-time nonprofit job, while Biff had remained a stay-at-home parent. He was the one who got up in the middle of the night when one of the kids had a bad dream or needed a glass of water. He was the one who made our meals, cleaned our house, did our laundry. These were things he'd realized over time that he was not only good at but also genuinely enjoyed (except for the laundry, which he hated). He maintained a high level of control over our household and had established a routine. Me asking him to have a baby meant that he was suddenly looking at also being the primary caretaker for a newborn on top of two elementary-age children who were still healing from the neglect they experienced before we came along. We'd finally reached a place of security and had established a secure rhythm in our lives, and I was asking him to toss it all out by introducing a new element. He was upset that I'd be carrying a baby he'd end up taking the larger share of responsibility for. In a word, he felt it was unfair, but like me, he was unable to express what he was feeling.

Pregnancy brain began to set in. I'd show up for a meeting at work and stand there as my staff stared at me, expectantly. "Oh, am I running this meeting?" I would ask. I couldn't give a good excuse for my airhead behavior either. I simply wasn't ready to tell them that their dude boss was pregnant and couldn't seem to figure out the best way to do it. Plus, maybe Biff was right. Maybe the first trimester *was* too early to tell anyone. In the first trimester, anything can happen.

CHAPTER SIX

HOW WE DO LOSS

—

The first pregnancy did not take.

Hailey didn't have school on the day of my follow-up ultrasound appointment, so we brought her to the doctor with us, telling her that I just needed a quick checkup. There was a small play area where we left her under the watchful eye of the receptionist, and Biff and I went back to the exam room, where I undressed and leaned back as the technician slathered cold jelly all over my belly.

There's a kids' book that we love, called *What Makes a Baby*, by Cory Silverberg and Fiona Smyth. In it, the author explains that an egg and sperm come together to make something that contains all the stories from each of their histories, and that sometimes, that tiny thing does not grow. Well, the tiny thing inside of me did not grow.

Before the appointment, Biff had actually seemed excited. He still hadn't been able to muster a lot of enthusiasm for the pregnancy but believed that hearing the heartbeat might finally jolt him out of his wariness. We watched on the monitor as the tech waved the wand over my belly and showed me where my uterus was, and then showed us a vague little shadow, saying "And now, here we can see the baby!"

Then it was silent. We all strained forward a bit, listening for a heartbeat, but the only noise I heard was the steady hum of the fluorescent lights above us.

"You know what?" the tech said, all smiles. "You just hold on for one second and I'll go get the doctor."

Biff and I looked at each other, and we just knew that something was wrong, but before we could say anything a doctor entered, chipper as the tech, and said, "Let's see what's going on here."

She repeated the wand movements and took some measurements. "Well, it only looks to be about four weeks along, so it's still a bit early yet."

"My hormone levels were at four weeks over two weeks ago," I said.

"Well, it's not always an exact science. Why don't you come back in another two weeks and we'll have another look. It might just be too early. It could be nothing."

I knew she was only trying to make us feel better, to give us a little bit of hope, but based on the last hormone test and how long my body had been feeling out of whack, I knew I had to have been six weeks at minimum and that if there wasn't a heartbeat then things weren't looking good. It was very much of one of those *Just give it to me straight, doctor!* moments. I knew the pregnancy was no longer happening for us, and I didn't need her coddling.

"If there's no heartbeat, I'm going to have a miscarriage, right?"

"Or the timing could just be off by a bit," she repeated. "But, yes, if you do end up miscarrying, I want you to come back and see me."

Since we had Hailey with us, we had zero time to process what we'd just learned and left the exam room with fake happy faces plastered on, my tummy still cold and sticky from the ultrasound gel. We kept up a steady stream of chatter on the way home, where a babysitter was watching Lucas.

That night I was hosting an event at the Q Center, Portland's LGBTQ resource hub. We had just enough time to grab Lucas and change clothes before heading over. I'd been leading a volunteer support program for LGBTQ prisoners for many years and had scheduled a holiday-card writing party to try and help spread some cheer to our members behind bars.

Biff tried to take me aside for a moment as we got ready, repeating the words the doctor had said, that maybe the first blood test had been off and we'd just miscalculated the dates.

"Stop," I said. "The pregnancy isn't happening, I'm going to miscarry, and it's fine. I guess my body's just broken."

I didn't mean that last part. Sometimes I go straight for gallows humor to get through tough moments, and I could tell Biff did not appreciate it at all. I'm usually the overly optimistic one, and the sudden role reversal in a situation that felt so extreme was jarring, but it was the only way I could process what was going on. My defense mechanisms had kicked in, not to mention that what was happening was to *my* body. Wasn't I allowed to deal with it however I wanted?

Biff drove with the kids to the Q Center, but I had to go pick up supplies, so I took the train. As I walked from the nearest commuter train stop to the Center, I began to feel a wetness in my underwear. *Shit.* I wasn't sure what was happening, but I thought that maybe this was it. This was the pregnancy, ending. I power-walked the final few blocks and was happy to see a healthy turnout of volunteers for the event; Biff and the kids were setting up tables and chairs, having already unpacked the boxes of holiday cards and pens. I told him I had to go to the bathroom, and when I did, sure enough, I was bleeding. I hadn't witnessed red spots in my underwear in over a decade. It was unsettling.

I didn't panic. I wasn't in any pain and there were no cramps, but I knew that I needed to find a pad, another scramble I hadn't experienced in twelve years. All of the bathrooms at the Q Center are gender neutral, but weirdly there were no menstrual supplies in the one I was in. I shoved some toilet paper into my underwear and ducked into the other bathroom to check. No luck. I snuck up to the reception area and whispered my request to the front desk volunteer, who rummaged through the desk drawers. Nothing there either.

I managed to find Stacey, a kind trans woman who was serving as executive director at the time. I knew that as a trans woman, she wouldn't question my need for a pad, so I asked if she knew where to find one. I heard Biff giving the group welcome in the other room as Stacey checked all the cabinets in the supply room. I was vaguely aware that I was abandoning Biff with a room full of volunteers and our children, but there wasn't much I could do. I could feel the blood getting thicker as it came out of me, and my desperation sharpened. "Ah! I know!" Stacey exclaimed. She shuttled me to the storage locker for the senior services program and snuck a Depends out of it. "I'm sorry we don't have anything else. I'm gonna add that to our order list right now," she said, her apology heightened by her soft Southern lilt. I thanked her profusely and snuck back into the bathroom.

I undressed myself from the bottom down, removing my shoes so I could dispose of my stained underwear completely. A rolling ache began to gather in my belly, like darkening clouds before a thunderstorm. I tried to hurry up, burying my bloody underwear in the trash can, awkwardly pulling on the senior diaper and my pants (and shoes!), then returning to the main room where the volunteers had begun introducing themselves. I apologized for my absence and asked for a moment alone with Biff.

"I'm having a miscarriage," I said quietly and calmly. "I'm starting to have a bit of pain and I can't stand up. I need you to run the event for me." The prisoner program had been my project for a long time, and Biff had only recently gotten involved, so this was a big ask—but I knew I had to tap out.

"Of course," he said. "What else can I do for you? Is there anything you need?"

"Nope, just want to get through this so we can go home. I'm sorry." I was sorry for not being able to stand up and present. I was sorry for not carrying our pregnancy to term. I was sorry for having the idea of a baby in the first place and for not knowing enough about biology to understand that I was already fertile and for stopping my hormones so early and for so many things. The ache swelled to become a pit of pain churning through my stomach and I doubled over, trying desperately to appear normal in what was a decidedly abnormal circumstance.

My seat was off to the side, and I watched Biff call everyone's attention back to the front of the room. He explained why we were doing the cards, reiterating how important it was for prisoners to feel connected to the outside world. He gave examples of the types of messages people could write in their letters. I heard him as if through a fog—the fog of pain, of loss, of shock that this was all happening so quickly. I tried to distract myself by critiquing Biff's speech and picturing how I would have phrased it differently. *You should say "prisoners," not inmates. You should say "prisons," not facilities. No one knows what "a facility" is.* Biff did a great job. I was just too out of it to see it.

I tried to seem normal, like this wasn't a big deal. But I could feel my uterus slowly evacuating the pregnancy into the Depends I was wearing. I felt compelled to stay in the room, carrying on like this wasn't happening. I'm usually a model of openness and authenticity, but this was not a situation I knew how to deal with. I couldn't believe my brilliant plan of having a baby was going so horribly wrong.

I decided to protect Biff from what I was experiencing so he wouldn't be scared to try again. I already knew that I was going to want to try to get pregnant again, preferably as soon as possible. This process was humbling, but my dream of having a baby didn't fade; if anything, it became stronger. Even though I had not exactly been excited about this pregnancy, I had still been looking forward to having a baby that was a little bit me and a little bit Biff and a little bit its own person. And I was terrified that once we got through this miscarriage ordeal, Biff was going to say something along the lines of, "Well, we tried for a pregnancy and this miscarriage thing was really hard to go through, so let's just forget it." When pulsating cramps began to course through my abdomen, I kept that same damn grin on my face, and when Biff came over to ask if I wanted to take a Lyft home, I reassured him that I was fine. "It's a little gross, that's all." He nodded and continued circulating through the room.

The event finally ended, and he packed everything up quickly, asking me what I needed once the room had emptied. I stood up carefully to make sure nothing was leaking, and mercifully there was no blood on my pants or the chair.

"Let's just get home. If you can hang with the kids that would be great, I just want to lie down for a bit. Maybe you can bring me some soup later if that's okay?"

What I wanted to say was, "I want you to hold me really close and tell me everything is going to be okay and that you're not going to give up on this," but I shut him out. That resolve strengthened once I got home and removed my clothes and the senior diaper. Thick dark blood poured out of me and I didn't know what to do. I sat on the toilet and tried to will the process forward, imagining the emptying of my uterus down the drain. The pain was acute now, having transitioned from rolling to stabbing, and I stopped myself from crying out just in time: I heard Biff's footsteps on the stairs to our room.

"Don't come up! I'm in the bathroom!"

I desperately wanted him to come up and hold my hand, but this was all so . . . yucky. I didn't want him to see me like this, doubled over on the toilet with blood coming out of me. This was not what he signed up for when he married me. I felt like there was this silent pact we had made when we first got together, though we had never said the words aloud: He agreed to marry a trans guy, and I agreed to never remind him that I'm actually a trans guy. This miscarriage seemed a violation of that agreement, which I had to contain as quickly as possible, or maybe our marriage would be over.

There was no need to protect myself from what was happening—I knew I was a man who could menstruate, get pregnant, and, yes, have a miscarriage. That part didn't bother me at all. It was just him I was trying to protect.

There seemed to be a lull in the bleeding, so I called down to Biff, asking him to come up with soup, if we had any. I rifled through the cabinet under the sink and found an old box of pads from when our friend Aimee had come to visit. By the time Biff made it back upstairs, I was peacefully lying in bed. He dropped off the soup and four ibuprofen and obeyed when I ushered him out of the room.

THE SUPPORT TEAM at the care clinic was wonderful. When I called to tell them the news, they transferred me to the nurse who had taken my vitals when I came in to be declared pregnant two weeks prior. She was calm and soothing, a welcome counter to my thin, shaky voice.

"This happens," she said in a practiced tone. "One in four known pregnancies isn't viable. And that's just the ones we know about. The rate is likely even higher."

I told her I knew that already. She sighed and proceeded haltingly, as if she wasn't sure this was the right thing to say.

"I'm going to tell you something that you might not be ready to hear. There will come a time, not today but at some point, when you will be grateful for this experience." I began to protest, but she continued. "It can seem like a miscarriage is a failure, but it is so, so not. It's the opposite. A miscarriage is a success. Trystan, your body recognized that this pregnancy wasn't viable—there's no way it would have become a baby. Your amazing body figured that out and took care of it, so that you would be healthy enough to get pregnant again. It did this so you can give birth to the next baby. Do you understand?" I nodded, though she couldn't see me through the phone. "Your body did exactly what it was supposed to do, and when you're ready I invite you to find that place where you can feel how miraculous that is. Your body is taking care of you. That's what this is—this is a success."

It was too much to take in all at once. I thanked her and hung up the phone, allowing the tears to fall.

I was feeling sad and gross and overwhelmed. I needed more support. Since I had locked Biff out of the experience completely, I went to Facebook. I posted a short message in the trans pregnancy group: "The pregnancy is over." Almost immediately my phone dinged with notifications. Other guys in the group were commenting with messages of love and support. Some shared stories of their own miscarriages, or the miscarriages of their partners or mothers. A few made comments along the lines of "I'm so sorry for your loss," and I immediately recoiled. I quickly discovered that I *hated* that sentiment.

I pulled up my original post and made a fast edit: "To clarify, I am sad that my pregnancy is over, but I do not see this as the loss of a baby or child. I see it as the loss of a potential future baby. I welcome all commiseration and advice, especially from those who have been in a similar situation. But please don't assume that I'm experiencing grief. Thank you all so much."

It's not that I wasn't experiencing grief—I was, in a way: grief that things were not going according to plan. Grief for the person I was before, a person who didn't know how much blood can come out of an uninjured human body. Grief for my relationship with Biff before I started this pregnancy process, a relationship that seemed so simple and sweet in retrospect, but which was now tarnished with this stain of bodily shame. Grief for the dark-eyed child that had visited me in my dreams. Yet it felt to me that she had simply returned to the ether, leaving us but not leaving the world, because she had never really been *in* it. What I was feeling was so complicated that it was infuriating to have others label it as a "loss." It was a rudimentary misunderstanding of what I was going through, and I hated it.

THE MISCARRIAGE ENDED UP lasting for weeks and into months. After the first few days of bleeding, a blood test revealed that the miscarriage had not fully finished on its own. I was instructed to "wait and see what happens," which meant that my body was not quite pregnant but not quite not-pregnant either. My chest was still swollen and tender, as it had been when I first suspected I was pregnant. My hips were still soft and wider than usual, and I had rolling cramps every few hours. During that time Biff was working at a mental health facility on the weekends. It was a 48-hour shift, and he slept on-site both Saturday and Sunday nights. I would drop off the kids at school every Monday and then drive out to pick him up. This meant I had the kids by myself all weekend, and I would often scramble to figure out how to entertain them while I was physically not at my best. In my attempt to find something easy and free for me and the kids to do on Sundays,

I found an earth-based church gathering with childcare and we began to go every week.

The pastor and I went to coffee one day, to get to know each other a little better. She was warm and thoughtful, and I liked her right away. She reminded me of Annie, who had officiated our wedding, and of the other spritely, heart-centered women I've been blessed to know throughout my life. She expressed genuine curiosity about our family. When she asked what I'd been looking for when I found her church, rather than tell her the story of needing free childcare, I found myself telling her a different story—a truer story.

"Honestly, I'm not a religious person. But I had just had a miscarriage and was looking for a space where I could try to make some meaning out of the experience."

Hm. Was that accurate? I knew immediately that it was. I had appreciated the quiet introspection offered by her service, and the loving space she created for deep contemplation. The rituals involving water and nature and letting go had brought me more comfort than I had been willing to examine. She let the silence stretch out between us before speaking.

"You had a miscarriage," she repeated, showing no visible reaction. "What was that like for you?"

The question was a revelation. *This* is what I had been wanting from others. No assumption about my experience. No forcing of sadness and loss. Simply openness and a willingness to listen, to hold the full complexity of my experience. I was overwhelmed with gratitude for her, and I shared with her the many nuances of what I was feeling—the trying to hide it all from Biff, the physical "yuck" of the blood and pain, the emptiness of feeling some ethereal spirit with me that was then suddenly gone. She gave me the gift I didn't know I needed. And I began to heal.

My body made that process difficult. It turns out I couldn't even miscarry right, and I ended up having to go through a D&C procedure in the hospital, where a doctor suctions out pregnancy tissue that hasn't successfully been cleared by the uterus on its own. The uncleared tissue was confusing my body into thinking it was still pregnant. I was trapped in this in-between space with my hormone levels all out of whack, nausea hitting at odd times, and the occasional leakage from my chest. Yet no fetus growing inside me. I was terrified about the procedure, having been told by a naturopath that it was invasive and painful, with terrible side effects. The naturopath told me that I should try to take expensive, unregulated herbs to encourage my body to clear the pregnancy on its own and I dutifully complied, but they didn't work and I had to go through with the procedure anyway. Everyone at the hospital was lovely, and within just a few hours the painless process was over. I rested for the afternoon and was feeling back to normal by the following day. Back to *normal* normal, like how I had felt before ever being pregnant at all. A blood test a few days later showed that the procedure was successful and I was officially no longer pregnant.

MY RELATIONSHIP WITH Biff became complicated and strange. I had pushed him away so effectively during the miscarriage that he had gotten used to focusing on Hailey and Lucas during the week, bringing me what I asked for when I was in pain, and working hard on the weekends. We fell into a fragile routine of sorts, like an old married couple with a tender shared history neither is willing to examine.

I knew that I wanted to try to get pregnant again, which is why I had been shielding him from the true horror of the miscarriage. I had scrubbed every drop of blood that had ended up on the bathroom floor, had taken every full pad out to the garbage bin myself, and had placed every phone call to the doctor in private so he wouldn't have to hear the gory details of my body's inner workings. I did it so he would be willing to try again. Preferably immediately. All of this was unspoken between us; I was too afraid to tell him my desires and aware that I would shatter if he didn't share them.

Then one day, as I was sitting on a bus headed from work to therapy, I received an email from him. The subject line read: "Thoughts." *Okay, here we go.*

Cut to five minutes later, and me on the bus reading this email and trying not to scream, my whole body shaking with fury and disappointment.

The email was long, but the main point was that he wanted us to wait a year before trying again, since we'd been living with so much chaos in our lives already. Out of all his carefully crafted words, these were the ones that leapt out at me: "I get that you think I might change my mind, but that's a risk I want you to take."

I knew—*just knew*—that he was ultimately going to back out of the plan but wanted to give me a little space first. *I'm being punished for miscarrying, and he's trying to trick me into believing there's still hope, when there isn't any. Wait a year? After all I've been through? A* year *?*

I seethed silently on the bus. I hit reply and began pounding out a response letting him know exactly where he could put his "thoughts." Once I had completed a perfect scathing takedown, I prepared to hit send but found my thumb hovering above the button, frozen. I suddenly remembered all the times I had taken action from a mental space of anger and hurt and disappointment. I thought about what it would be like to respond rather than react. And, perhaps most importantly, I tried to remember what my end goal was. At first, I thought that it was to have a baby. That's what I ultimately wanted. But upon further reflection, I realized that my end goal was not to have a baby. It was to be with Biff. He was, after all, the love of my life. Had I been letting my short-term dream of a baby drown out my long-term dream of staying married, in love, and happy?

I took a deep breath and saved the email as a draft. I pulled the wire to notify the bus driver that I was getting off and took some time to walk around downtown Portland. I needed to get my head right. I called my friend Heather and asked for her take on things.

"At the end of the day, do you trust Biff or not?" she asked me. And of course, I told her I did. Unequivocally. In fact, there were so many times when I had wanted to do something and he had talked me out of it, and I was grateful. Like telling the kids I was pregnant—I couldn't imagine what they would have experienced if they truly knew why Daddy was upstairs in bed for almost a full week. I didn't think they could possibly see the miscarriage as anything other than a baby dying. Their sibling—dying. They had been through more than enough, and Biff was right to protect them from the process. I did trust him. After speaking with Heather, I went to my actual therapy appointment and managed to put myself in order mentally.

Several hours later I returned home to Biff. Instead of responding to him via email, I spoke to him directly. We put a movie on for Hailey and Lucas and I sat with him on our bed.

"I love you," I told him. "And I love you more than I love the idea of having a baby. If you think we should wait, we should wait. And if you don't think we should do this at all . . . then we shouldn't do it. At the end of the day, I trust you and your judgment. And if I have to choose between you and a baby, I choose you."

Biff sat in stunned silence. Clearly he had been expecting a major showdown. When he finally spoke, he said, "What did your therapist do to you?!" We laughed, and I told him she didn't do anything—I just loved him so much and didn't ever want to do anything that might compromise our life together. I was willing to let go of anything to make us work.

He reassured me that he wasn't giving up on the idea of a baby, but just wanted to let things settle down a bit for us as a family. My stomach in knots, I told him I understood and would wait as long as he wanted.

Two weeks later, he asked if I was ready to start trying. "I know it's hard for you to be off your hormones, and it's stupid to make you keep waiting. Let's just do it. Let's make a baby."

IT'S NOT LOST on me that by finally backing off from my wish for Biff to actively champion us having a baby, I ended up getting exactly that. Sometimes letting go of a fixed belief allows the emergence of something much more powerful than what you even first imagined. Biff began to talk about how cool it would be to experience parenthood through a lens that wasn't so dependent on the American court system, and he started coming home with adorable little baby outfits that he'd stash in our dresser: a onesie with a seahorse on it, tiny rainbow leggings, a striped cap.

His baby fever finally equaled mine, and six months later I was pregnant again.

Notes from Life in Our Family

Get Comfortable (with Discomfort).

There will inevitably be times when you and your partner don't agree. Biff decidedly did not want a baby, and I did. We had to live in that space of disagreement for quite a while, but we were used to it. We hadn't agreed on how to view his family or whether to move to Portland or when to adopt the kids. We were practiced in disagreement. We were comfortable with it.

One way we make our way through disagreement is to remember that it is okay to disagree. This may be a controversial statement. As I write this in 2021, it has become accepted to shame and bully those who have a different opinion. But your relationship is not Twitter. No one is obligated to pile onto anyone else—you can hear your partner's opinion, respect it, and not agree. It can be uncomfortable to sit in that disagreement, but life is not a zero-sum game. You don't have to be right all the time. You can choose to be in relationship instead, and decide not to fight.

Of course, some disagreements cannot be lived with (like when one person wants a baby and the other doesn't). You can love your partner very much while also wholeheartedly disagreeing with their point of view. There will have to be compromise somewhere; one of you will have to give.

Get Supportive.

Only after my miscarriage did I learn that it has been so taboo in our culture that those who experience it often aren't given the room and support they need to process through it. When we hear of a miscarriage, many of us (especially those in the feminist, therapeutic, and birthing world) have been taught to say, "I'm sorry for your loss."

A word of caution: Just as it's wrong to assume a pregnancy loss isn't a big deal, it's just as wrong to assume that it is! When you're supporting someone through any complicated life experience, try asking them: "What was that like for you?"

I first heard this from a gifted pastor, and it has come in handy many times in the years since. When a friend's abusive parent dies: "What was that like for you?" When someone shares that they got divorced: "What was that like for you?" When someone decides that transitioning isn't for them: "What was that like for you?"

It's simple, open, curious, and loving. Allow those around you to name their own experiences first, then support them based on their response.

Get Supported.

Be careful who you ask for support. I was so desperate for help during my pregnancy and miscarriage that I allowed a lot of people into my orbit, including those with their own agenda.

I was terrified about my D&C procedure because I had let a naturopath put that fear into me, which ended up being unfounded.

If you're not getting support that feels like it's helping you, run. If you're experiencing judgment, fear-based advice, or anything that doesn't seem to be true (though it may feel real to the person giving it), run.

In the pregnancy and birth world, there are so many opinions and different ways of approaching things, which is fine. But a lot of those ways come with an agenda and may not work for you. You're not obligated to do what people tell you to, or to believe what they believe. It's okay to decide not to follow them.

The stakes feel so high when we're dealing with the creation of a new life, and the bringing of that new life into the world, but don't let anyone take advantage of your tenderness around it. Do what feels empowering to you, ask for advice from people you trust, and be ready to confidently tell people to fuck off if they try to shame you for your decisions.

CHAPTER SEVEN

HOW WE DO PREGNANCY

——

After all the drama with the miscarriage, Biff and I tried for several months to conceive and timed everything out. It wasn't working and it wasn't working until it finally worked. And this time, when I peed on the stick and the plus sign appeared, I cried out of joy and relief and surprise. I had been neurotically monitoring my cycle and didn't think we had timed things accurately that month. In fact, "getting pregnant" was less fun than it sounded, and scheduled sex was feeling more like a chore than a way to connect with Biff and create new life. I had decided to switch things up a bit and surprised him one night at his job for a secret rendezvous in the bathroom (a major feat considering I had to hire a babysitter to pull the whole thing off). Apparently that furtive tryst did the trick, and I was finally, officially, knocked up.

WE HAD STARTED DROPPING HINTS to the kids that we wanted to have a baby.

Hailey was six when we first started talking to her about being a big sister at some point. One night, when I was tucking her in, she asked if I "really, actually" wanted to have a baby. I tried to sound nonchalant and dismissed the question with a breezy "Oh, I don't know, honey. Maybe!" But she pressed on. "No, Daddy, you *do* know," she declared. "Yes or no, do you want to have a baby?" I sighed and sat down on the bed. "Yes, honey. I do want to have a baby." She promptly burst into tears. "But you already have a baby. And it's me!"

Over time, though, both kids softened to the idea. We even started brainstorming baby names together. Lucas still wasn't excited, per se, but he wasn't showing as much blatant distress as Hailey had during that first conversation. In fact, Hailey had started to proactively ask about when a baby might come. She already knew many men and non-binary people who had given birth, so the idea of me getting pregnant wasn't that new or different to her.

After the first burst of joy and excitement, I settled into pregnant life. We quietly went to doctor's visits and ultrasounds, and I managed the first-trimester nausea without the kids catching on. We weren't sure that this pregnancy would take, so I only told my very closest friends and my trans pregnancy community on Facebook. We proceeded with caution, having learned that, for us, pregnancy loss would be better handled with a small group of people. The first few months were blissfully uneventful. When I hit week thirteen (aka the second trimester), we decided it was time to officially tell the kids.

We planned a nice family dinner at home. Biff bought sparkling cider and I made a copy of the ultrasound photo to show them. We thought through how we would approach the situation, discussing it as an opportunity to be a big sister, for Hailey, and an opportunity to be given more freedom and independence, for Lucas. The day of our announcement came, and we all sat down to one of the kids' favorite dishes. As we poured the cider into plastic champagne flutes, an excited Hailey (who loves anything sweet) slowly narrowed her eyes in suspicion.

"Wait a minute," she said, turning her head to face Biff. "What are we celebrating?" Biff and I made eye contact and sat down, reaching across the table to grasp each of our children's hands in our own. Biff began.

"Well—Hailey, Lucas . . . we wanted to let you guys know that—" He paused for dramatic effect as I pulled out the ultrasound photo. "We're having a baby!" he exclaimed as I showed them both the photo. We had expected Hailey to react badly, given her previous animosity toward the whole baby idea. But much to our surprise, she jumped out of her chair with joy, screaming at the top of her lungs. "I'm going to be a big sister! I'm going to be a big sister! Where will it sleep? Can I choose the name? When will I be old enough to babysit?"

Lucas rolled his eyes and slumped in his chair. "Great. A loud, screaming baby. My dad is pregnant. Awesome."

We tried to hold space for both reactions, appreciating Hailey for her excitement but reminding her that Lucas doesn't like loud noises, so she needed to control her excitement. And we told Lucas that we would do the best job we could at keeping the baby from crying too much, but that babies cry when they need something so yes, the baby would cry on occasion, maybe even often, depending on its personality.

"And we know that it's not every day that a man gets pregnant, so we will leave it up to you to decide if and when you tell your friends, okay?" Lucas immediately began to tell us that he wanted us to keep it a secret entirely, requesting that he be able to tell his friends that the baby is his cousin or a baby we were babysitting. Biff and I glanced at each other in frustration. We had known that this wouldn't be easy but hadn't anticipated that Lucas would be so distraught that he would ask us to lie about the whole process. Biff took over.

"Lucas, no. We will not be dishonest about who this baby is. Everyone will know that the baby is your little sibling. That will be totally clear. You can't ask us to lie, because it doesn't make sense. And Lucas, you know that all your friends already know we're gay and we're your dads, right? It's very obvious, despite what you told Halil last week," Biff said, referring to a conversation we'd had with Lucas's teacher, during which she informed us that she'd overheard Lucas telling his friend

Halil that Biff was his uncle and I was Biff's roommate. I cut in, trying to keep things from escalating.

"Hey, okay. We can't lie about the baby, but is there anything else we *can* do so you know you're in charge of your part of this story?" He paused, thinking it over. Hailey tried to interrupt with her own ideas, as usual, but I put my hand out to stop her. "Let him think and decide for himself, Hailey." Finally, he spoke, looking at Biff.

"Okay. What if, I don't want Daddy to come to pick me up at school when he's like, really, really pregnant." Biff, exasperated, began to cut him off.

"Lucas, Daddy doesn't even pick you up from school. I do! This is—" but I interjected again, speaking directly to Lucas.

"That's fine, buddy. I'm happy to either cover up when I pick you up from school or have Dada do it after I start really showing. Okay? Anything else?" I wanted to really hear him through this process, because so little is really in kids' control, and feeling powerless is its own kind of hurt.

"Yes," he stated, directing his gaze at Hailey. "I don't want *her* telling all of my friends all of my business all the time!" He stood up and started breathing faster, his face reddening. "She always tells everyone all about our life, 'Oh, I have two dads and a mom that couldn't take care of me,' when I want to keep some things PRIVATE."

At this point, Hailey stood up, too, saying, "I'm PROUD of my sweet daddies and my nice life and I can tell whoever I want about it!"

Biff and I looked at each other as the kids continued to yell about who was allowed to say what to whom at what time. Resigned, we clinked our glasses together and had a sip of cider.

"Well, I think it's safe to say we 'nailed it!' with this announcement," I said sarcastically over the din of fighting. Biff smirked as I turned back to the kids and asked them to settle down.

"Okay, okay, okay. Lucas, I hear you saying that you would like to decide when and how to tell your school friends, is that right?"

"Yes, and HAILEY—" he tried to continue, pointing her way.

"Aah!" I stuck my hand out, finger up. The universal sign for "You're done talking and I'm in charge here." He quieted down. I turned to Hailey.

"And I hear *you* saying that you would like to be able to tell your school friends whenever and however you would like. Is that right?" Hailey, who had learned her lesson watching my interaction with Lucas, simply nodded her head once while glaring Lucas's way.

"Okay!" I declared. "Lucas, you may tell your friends however you like. You may *not* lie about this baby or this pregnancy, but you don't have to tell anyone if you don't want to. You are also not allowed to tell Hailey that she can't tell her friends or try to make her feel bad about telling her friends. Good?" I asked for his assent with a thumbs-up, which was still our universal sign for checking in. He nodded his head resolutely, thumbs-up. I turned to Hailey.

"Hailey!" I tried to mimic the same tone I had directed at Lucas, adding a little silliness to the conversation. "You may tell your friends however you like. You may *not* tell Lucas's friends, or try to make him feel bad about wanting to keep parts of his life private. He has a right to do that. Good?" I raised my eyebrows and held my thumb up, and she giggled and put her thumb up in response.

"Good," I stated firmly as I poured everyone more apple cider and we continued with dinner. The kids had more questions, most disturbingly the one in which Hailey asked how I got pregnant. I addressed that question by explaining: "Well, just like in the book, in order to make a baby, you need sperm, an egg, and a place for the baby to grow. Dada has the sperm and I have the egg. I also have the uterus, which is where the baby will grow."

Her brow furrowed as she tried to understand. "So, Dada took his sperm and gave it to your egg?" she inquired. I nodded delicately. She looked at Biff for her next question: "Did it hurt, getting the sperm out of your body?" He shook his head no. Satisfied, she began asking what we were going to be having for dessert. Biff and I looked at each other and sighed. We could keep coasting by on the sex question, answering only and exactly what she asked and not being forced to talk about intercourse at all. Whew.

HAILEY AND LUCAS both recognized that this would be a unique situation in their school community. None of their school friends' parents were transgender; there weren't any other gay dads at their school either. But we were fairly certain they wouldn't experience any trouble from their peers once everyone found out.

"Today for show and tell, I brought in this! It looks blurry a little bit, that's because it is, but it is called an 'ultrasound.' It's a special kind of picture of a baby in a belly and it's my little baby sister. Or brother. Or . . . sibling." Yes, Hailey decided to bring an ultrasound into her classroom to tell her friends that she was going to be a big sister. Given that she was in second grade, we weren't sure how it would go, but as a precocious child she was unlikely to listen to our warnings about transphobia anyway, so we gave her our blessing. When she came from school, I asked her how it went.

"Great!" she said. "Everyone is really excited for me and helped me think of some baby names, if you were planning to let *me* name the baby."

"Um . . . we weren't, but I would love to hear them." She began to rattle off the names she and her classmates had come up with ("Chestnut, Walnut, pretty much anything with 'nut' is gonna be good"), and I chuckled in disbelief at how charmed her life with us in Portland was. So many of the trans men I'd connected with online had shared stories of their kids being tormented by peers and even school staff when stories of their pregnancies had surfaced. I wasn't sure if it was Hailey's charm or our liberal school community, but I appreciated how well things were going for her. The next day, though, when she came home from school, she said that things had changed.

"Everyone was super mean today," she shared. "Sara said that her dad told her that boys couldn't have babies so I must be lying. And Xian says that his mom said I was wrong or didn't understand what I was saying because only girls can have babies. I told them they were both wrong because my dad is transgender and used to be a girl and still has some parts of a girl's body so he *can* have a baby, but they were all really confused." I gave her a hug, but she shrugged me off. "Whatever, I'm still happy about a baby and it doesn't matter what their parents say about us. Can I go play now?" I told her she could, and she skipped off to her room. A few minutes later I heard her talking to herself in different voices, pretending to be a dog and a cat playing astronauts (or something like that).

"Nothing fazes that kid," Biff said that night when I recounted the story, shaking his head in disbelief. While very sensitive to others' emotions, Hailey was perpetually unperturbed by the actions and options of others. She would cry at the drop of a hat, especially if she had experienced any measure of physical discomfort (stubbed toe, bumping into a chair, *almost* bumping into a chair), and if anyone else was upset or hurt, she would cry for them too. But when it came to her own emotional sensitivity, it just seemed to be ironclad. When the rare occasion of teasing came up, she would shrug her shoulders and dismiss it. Considering how deeply it hurt me when Lucas showed shame and embarrassment about having two dads as his parents, I was in awe of Hailey's confidence and resilience. *How do I get to be like that?* I still haven't figured it out.

THE THOUGHT OF A NEW BABY continued to challenge Lucas's sense of security. One day he was being particularly grumpy, stomping around the house and calling everyone names. Frustrated, I closed my eyes and took a deep breath, vowing to respond constructively even though I did not feel at all interested in dealing with his stuff. I walked over to him and knelt down so we would be eye to eye.

"Lucas, what's going on with you? Can you tell me why you're upset?"

This tiny amount of compassion broke the attitude bubble and he burst into tears, his little-kid face suddenly red and wet. He struggled to catch his breath and we had to just stay there for a moment, with me modeling big, obvious in-and-out breathing until he mirrored me and steadied himself enough to speak.

"I'm just scared that you will love the baby more than you love me, because the baby came out of your body and I didn't." He collapsed into me and I held him for a long time. I had been expecting this concern and had practiced what I would say. Because this fear isn't a silly one! It makes perfect sense that an adopted kid would have this worry, and I wanted to provide him with something he could hold on to and come back to later on, when his insecurities crept up again.

When he was ready, I pulled away from him and looked into his eyes. "Lucas . . . this baby, whoever it turns out to be, is totally random. I don't know him! He's just like, a mix of me and Dada. That's it. But *you* are special. We knew you when you became our family. We *chose* you. Okay? We chose you." I let him sit with that for a moment, and it did seem to speak to the part of him that was feeling most afraid. I reminded him that we could have this conversation again anytime he wanted to, and we shared a big hug. I took more deep breaths, hoping that we were doing the right thing.

LUCAS'S INSECURITIES ABOUT HIS VALUE in our family were just the beginning of the onslaught of opinions about my pregnancy. One day, around eighteen weeks in, I came home from work and found Biff upstairs in our bedroom.

"Have you seen this interview?" I asked him, holding out my phone with a top-tier morning show host and famous Black transgender actress visible on the screen, sitting across from each other in an interview. Biff squinted his eyes like he does when looking at something detailed, and nodded his head yes.

"That's from like, two years ago, isn't it?" he asked.

"Sure, but I just watched it again on the bus and it still pisses me off. How come we're making Black trans women have these hard conversations on TV and then there's people like you and me just, like, living in Portland reaping the cultural rewards?"

I shook my head warily. "It just doesn't seem fair or right."

Biff shrugged. "Okay, well then *you* go on TV and talk about being a pregnant man and answer those stupid questions. God knows you've got enough support around you, compared to so many other trans people."

It was supposed to be just another tiny exchange between us, one of hundreds we have every week: me bringing something up, us discussing it a bit, then both of us moving on. Only, I couldn't move on. I tossed and turned at night, thinking about it. Laverne Cox, Janet Mock, Carmen Carrera . . . all of these amazing trans women of color, working tirelessly to push the culture forward by telling their stories and putting themselves out there again and again. For years, whenever a microphone was shoved in my face, I got out of the way so a trans woman could speak into it. If I was invited to speak at a conference or rally or vigil, I respectfully declined, offering the names of trans women who could speak instead. Because transphobia impacts trans women so much more than it impacts trans men (and with such fiercer brutality), trans men often know that it is our job to center their voices and experiences. It's no accident that there are so many famous trans women and so few famous trans men—we, in the trans movement, planned it that way.

But I never really thought through what comes after that. I never imagined that it would *work*, and that trans women's voices—trans women of color in particular—would ring out with such clarity and vision that they would end up shouldering the entire burden of cultural change for the trans movement. And now, with trans women answering questions about their anatomy on television, it just felt icky. I spent days feeling entirely distant from everything around me, watching my dreamy life as an outsider might: my safe Portland community, my colorful house and gregarious friends, and my sweet, beautiful family. What price had I paid for this idyllic life? What right did I have to this bliss, when so many others were being fed into the churn of media clickbait? A slow, steady drumbeat began to emerge from my psyche. It wasn't right—it wasn't fair—for me to have all of this while expecting others to do the hard work of changing hearts and minds. Especially when my entire professional life had been dedicated to changing hearts and minds.

Days after that initial conversation, I sat across from Biff at the tiny bar by our house, having bribed Hailey and Lucas to stay home so the two of us could have a quick-and-dirty date night. Biff had red wine and I had a soda, and after a discussion about setting up the baby's room, I told him that I thought we should tell our story publicly. I explained all of the considerations I'd been mulling over, about our obligation to be part of the cultural story about queerness and family and trans rights. I could tell that he didn't "get it."

"Sounds dangerous to me, but you're the trans one here and it's your pregnancy. Ultimately, it's up to you." And so it was (sort of) decided: I would go public with my/our story. It seemed so simple at the time: sharing the burden of trans education with others in the community. Using the "hook" of a pregnant man to start a larger conversation about trans rights and families. That night I reached out to *The Longest Shortest Time*, with the subject line: "I have news." The email had just one sentence: "I'm pregnant." I was excited to tell this part of my story, imagining the same listeners that heard our adoption story might be interested to hear the next chapter. *Maybe a few hundred people will hear it*, I thought. *That should help change people's minds.*

It was a simpler time. A more naive time. I had no idea that my life was about to split into two distinct parts: before becoming "the pregnant man," and after.

THOUGH THE SECOND TRIMESTER was medically very easy for me (I got the famed boost in energy), I was likely the most annoying patient my providers ever had. I was completely obsessed with learning everything I could about pregnancy. Not only was I reading dozens of books about it, but I was also spending all of my free time reading blogs and scrolling through pregnancy posts in Facebook groups. My platform was growing bigger and bigger as the days passed. First, there was the podcast interview, which quickly became one of the most popular episodes released by the show. Then *Cosmopolitan* magazine posted about it and the UK tabloids followed suit. Within a matter of hours, news outlets across the globe were covering my story and I was dealing with an onslaught of media attention. The trouble with the single-story narrative is that one person ends up representing all people in their community. It became clear to me that my pregnancy had to go perfectly, or everyone in the world would point at me and say, "See? This is why *these people* shouldn't be allowed to have children." It was an enormous amount of pressure, and I wanted to do right by my community. I knew, now that my story was out there, that I was representing all transgender parents everywhere, and I simply had to Get It Right.

At every wellness appointment, I subjected my midwife to a barrage of questions. Week 6: "Am I gaining enough weight?" "Am I gaining too much weight?" Week 12: "It says online that I should exercise, but also that I shouldn't exercise too much. How far should I be walking each day? Is swimming okay? How long should I swim for?" Week 18: "I read somewhere that I shouldn't have *any* alcohol, but another source said a little is okay? Can I have one sip of Biff's wine or no?" "You mentioned that I can have one cup of coffee a day. How much caffeine is safe, because different coffees have different levels of caffeine in them so 'one cup' isn't really a precise recommendation."

Poor woman.

I also demanded to have an ultrasound at every appointment. Again, I know this must have seemed high maintenance, but I was receiving hundreds of messages on social media every single day, telling me that I was going to give birth to a monster. Even though rationally I knew that they were wrong, I still wanted to see the fetus anytime I could. Having been a transgender person in this world, I've been told in many ways that my body is disgusting, that nothing good will ever happen to me. These strangers, whether they knew it or not, were tapping into my deepest, most strongly held beliefs—that I am unworthy of love. No amount of reassurance from my beloveds has ever been able to touch those deep wounds; I have been forced to live alongside them and may die with them still unresolved. And so, I wanted those ultrasounds.

In retrospect, I could have just told the midwife that I was being harassed by hundreds of strangers on the internet and needed reassurance that my pregnancy was going well, but I couldn't get those words out of my mouth at the time. I was in full-on survival mode, managing interview requests, getting feedback on my media appearances from trans messaging professionals, and generally trying not to make things worse by bungling this opportunity. Oh, and also growing a human being inside of my torso.

Once I hit 32 weeks, Biff and I were supposed to go to a birthing class sponsored by my insurance carrier. We only made it to the first session, because it was so awkward. We were the only two-man couple in the whole group, which quickly sorted itself into "mommy teams" and "daddy teams." Even though my therapist had called ahead to work with the instructor on being inclusive, and even though the instructor had really done her best, it was just too weird for us. We skipped out on the second class, opting instead to spend the day at the annual Trans March surrounded by our community as we mentally prepared to welcome a child into the world. At the march, I overheard a tourist walk by and say, "That's a pregnant man." The whole world was, both literally and figuratively, gawking at me.

It was a lot.

THEN THINGS STARTED to get dark. If you're a transgender person, you might want to skip to page 150. The
every-once-in-awhile message of disgust from strangers quickly
became a torrent of negativity. Every buzz of my phone brought
a new level of nastiness—someone else calling me "a fucking
cancer on this planet" and "a disgusting circus freak." People
told me that they felt sorry for my children, that they were
going to call child protective services to have Hailey and Lucas
taken away, that my baby was going to be born deformed.
"That poor child," was a common refrain in the comments
section.

At first, I thought I could handle it. I had been living as
a transgender man for over a decade at that point; much of
that time had been spent talking to homophobic strangers
about LGBTQ rights. *I'm strong*, I told myself. *They can't hurt
me.* Boy was I wrong. Yes, I had been face-to-face with voters
who told me that they didn't believe I should be able to get
married, that being gay was against their beliefs, and that they
didn't think transgender people needed to be protected from
discrimination. But this was entirely different. This was not
polite, reasoned discourse. This was not connecting with, and
even disagreeing with, sane and rational human beings. This
was, as Biff put it, "some next-level shit."

I fought with my own stubbornness. It felt weak to give in and
admit that I just couldn't show up for this toxicity. That maybe I

should stay away from the internet for a while. That social media had become a disgusting stew of judgment and shame. Even when a friend posted something nice about me, the first comment was usually something awful: "This is fake news! That's not a pregnant man! That's just a really ugly, hairy woman!" I couldn't even find the supportive messages because they became mixed up in everything else. And I couldn't look away.

The human brain is hardwired to look for threats everywhere—and it perceives any threat to oneself at the same level as the threat posed by a tiger or an earthquake. I'm sure that the negative comments were vastly outweighed by the positive ones—and I really did try to take in the positive ones while ignoring the negative. But I just couldn't do it. My eyes slid past the "Good for him!" and "This is so cool!" comments and got stuck on the "LOLOLOL" and puking emojis. On a deep level, I was terrified. Now the whole world could see what I already knew: I'm crazy. No one will ever love me. I'm not really a man. I don't deserve to be happy.

I stopped sleeping entirely.

Whenever I started drifting off, I found myself wracked with violent nightmares about giving birth to a bat, a pterodactyl, a snake. One night I jerked awake and just sobbed, letting out all the darkness that was pent up inside of me. Biff woke up to me shaking and sleepily asked what was wrong.

"They hate us," was the only thing I could say. "They hate us."

After all of the advocacy I had done to change laws and

policies, educating employers and teachers and business own-
ers, I had never truly grasped the level of transphobia that
existed in the world. And I was ashamed that it had taken me so
long to wake up to it. *This* is what my trans women friends had
spent years yelling about. It's not that I hadn't believed them
when they told me stories of victimization and violence; I did!
But I didn't viscerally understand their experiences until the
full weight of this hatred was directed at me, and I completely
caved beneath it.

Meanwhile, I was engaged in a long and protracted battle
against my body and the medical systems I was trapped in. As
I slogged into week 37 of the pregnancy, I faced ever-increasing
pain. A prenatal chiropractor informed me that I had "rib separation," which is exactly what it sounds like: The fetus was so
big that my ribs were pulling away from my sternum and spine.
Every time I took a breath, my ribs expanded a little more, tug-
ging themselves out of the protective cartilage that held them in
place. I thought back to the sunny, long-haired doulas on You-
Tube who had blithely repeated the phrase: "A body can't grow
a baby that's too big for it."

False. A body *can* grow a baby that's too big for it. And that's
what was happening with me. As the fetus grew larger and larger
and the toll it was taking on my body grew worse and worse, I
calculated all possible scenarios and determined that a medical induction would be the safest, most controlled labor process,
unfolding under the watchful eye of medical experts who had
seen hundreds of births over the years. For those not in the world

of childbirth, induction is the process of encouraging a pregnant body to go into labor. No one truly knows what triggers the body to start the process of labor on its own—some say it's a chemical released when the fetus's lungs are fully developed, but that's never been proven. A medical induction usually happens at a hospital and involves a series of medical interventions (including an injection of a hormone called Pitocin) designed to inspire the body's natural labor processes. That's what I wanted. I wanted to be mere feet from someone who went to medical school. I wanted to be able to see the fetus's heartbeat on the screen, to see my own contractions displayed clearly above my bed, to feel connected to the process through these technologies. That's what made me feel safest and most empowered when I visualized my labor.

AS MY MEDICAL SITUATION DETERIORATED around week 38, my story had gone more than viral. At this point, I had been featured in an article on CNN and on the front page of the *Washington Post*'s website. French journalists had flown to Portland to take our photo and interview us for *Paris Match* (which is akin to *People* magazine, only French). A Spanish documentarian spent a weekend with us and released a special about our family. My pregnancy had officially become a Big Deal. This fame (or infamy, perhaps) continued to be a double-edged sword. While we had reached our intended goals of increasing the visibility of transgender men and sparking a larger cultural conversation about transgender people and families, it had also resulted in my life being turned upside down as a toxic slurry of transphobia rolled over me, again and again. I had wanted to stop doing interviews altogether, but Biff reminded me that once a story is on the internet, it's there forever. "The trolls don't stop just because you do," he rightly said. "The only thing that happens is that they get to own the story instead of you." So, I barreled onward. I avoided comments sections entirely, and my friends volunteered to run my social media pages so I wouldn't have to read the worst of the backlash. But even as protected as I was, I quickly realized that the scrutiny wasn't going to end when my pregnancy did; just as the pregnancy process had to go perfectly, the birth process had to go perfectly as well.

I begged the obstetrics office to let me come in and see the midwife who had been treating me. I brought her a stack of studies showing the many times that researchers had found induction to be perfectly safe if no other issues had arisen during the pregnancy. I knew in my bones that this fetus was fully cooked and was ready to make its appearance. But the midwife shook her head and reminded me that "the discomfort of a pregnant person is not grounds for induction."

Sitting on that exam table while I was told that no, they would not induce me—*could* not induce me before 40 weeks ("it's against policy")—is still one of the most gut-wrenching moments of my life. I felt totally and utterly powerless at the hands of this medical machinery that refused to listen to what I wanted to do with my own body. As the midwife left the exam room, I turned to Biff and burst into tears. Breathing was hard.

Sleeping was impossible. I wanted to not be pregnant anymore, and I was willing to do anything to get it over and done with.

The midwife had mentioned that I could "maybe try acupuncture?" So I scheduled some acupuncture sessions and reached out to the naturopath I knew, to see if there were any other ways I could get an induction process started on my own. "One to three droppers of black cohosh under the tongue, and don't let them induce you until you're at 43 weeks or more. Pitocin is poison," they said.

Desperate to be done with pregnancy, I did what the naturopath said. I went to an herb shop in Portland and found black cohosh. I took one to three droppers full as suggested. I sat through painful sessions of acupuncture several times. A loving friend of my sister's gifted me his sessions in a salt float tank, and those hours in sensory deprivation were the only pain-free ones I had in those final weeks of pregnancy. In that warm, dark room, weightless in the water, I practiced self-hypnosis, getting ready for labor and begging aloud for this baby to just be born already. "We are so excited to meet you, whenever you want to come out!" I told it gently. Other times I was more insistent: "Please come out. I don't know how much longer I can do this."

I took long walks, as suggested by the naturopath, and ate spicy food. Other than the occasional contraction (which is a normal part of late pregnancy and not an indicator of labor), nothing happened. When the naturopath recommended castor oil, I stopped to evaluate the situation further. I began

researching the academic literature on blue and black cohosh.
What I found was a whole lot of nothing. There has never been
a single study that shows that any herbal induction methods
work. In fact, I found that there are more instances of people
becoming mortally ill from attempting induction than there are
instances of people experiencing labor more quickly. Reading
these studies, I started to panic. I examined the bottle of black
cohosh I had purchased, searching the label for any information on the concentration or strength of the tincture. It wasn't
there. In fact, the label didn't even tell me where or when the
herb had been collected or processed.

Wait a minute, I thought, incredulously. *One to three droppers
full? That's either one dose . . . or three doses. Of something that's
never been proven to do what I want it to do. That was made in a
location I don't know anything about. That has never been tested by
an outside organization or trusted person.* I put the bottle down
and started to panic. *What am I doing?* It seemed that everyone
around me had an agenda of their own, with little regard for
what I—a living, breathing, birthing person—actually wanted.
I had been banging on the iron door of a broken medical system
while also putting god-only-knows-what into my body, which
was going straight into the bloodstream of my developing baby.

"This ends now," I declared as I threw the black cohosh into
the trash and picked up the phone. No one was going to control
this part of my pregnancy but me. I called the OB. I was not
going to be pregnant a single day longer, and that was final.

✳

Notes from Life in Our Family

Get Educated.

What do you need to feel great about your pregnancy? Or if "great" is too strong a word, what do you need to feel okay about your pregnancy? What would an empowered pregnancy look like for you? For me, it meant being able to see the fetus at every medical checkup. It meant going to see my provider as often as possible so I could be reassured that everything was okay. It meant asking if therapy was included in my insurance and asking enough times for them to actually help me schedule an appointment. It also meant copy-pasting pregnancy articles into a Word document and re-gendering all of the pronouns so I could send Biff information on what I was experiencing without him having to read "she" and "her" everywhere. Think through what you need to feel good and ask for it. I do it as politely (and firmly!) as possible, but everyone has their own style. Find yours and use it!

Get Uncomfortable.

The question of how we talk to the kids about sex and pregnancy is a tough one, and the science on how kids best learn about sex is still evolving. In our family, we talk to the kids about this topic the same way we talk to them about anything: in short, developmentally appropriate conversations peppered throughout all aspects of their lives. Luckily, neither Biff nor I have many hang-ups about sex and sexuality, which is surprising, since he was raised in an Evangelical household and I was raised in a family where we almost never talked about sex either, but for our own reasons that weren't religious. I'm not sure how he and I ended up being comfortable with our bodies and their capacity for pleasure, but talking about sex and relationships and romance and consent has always come naturally for us both as parents.

Because we are queer, the conversations about sex have always been completely separate from the conversations about procreation, which is how I think it should be. Sex often *is* for pleasure, and a good chunk of procreation doesn't involve sex. Try to be honest with kids without oversharing, giving enough to help them navigate early childhood and avoid being victimized, knowing that our primary job is to ensure that they're kept safe.

CHAPTER EIGHT

HOW WE DO BIRTH

———

"All right, it'll be time to push in about ten minutes," said the nurse with the British accent.

PUSH? Oh shit. I forgot to plan for pushing!

I remembered a book that had come in the mail, *Prepare to Push,* by Kim Vopni, all about the actual act of childbearing. I hadn't read it. There had been too many other things to do! Too many other books to read! Why hadn't I read that book?! I was not prepared to push.

Then I flashed back to the delivery classes we were supposed to attend. Maybe if we had attended the second session I would have learned about the pushing part. After I spoke with the doctor, begging him to schedule my induction, everything is blurry in my memory. When people ask me how exactly I gave birth, I often use a beloved phrase to describe it: "gradually, then suddenly."

I FELT TERRIBLE going above my midwife's head, but I was done. I was at exactly thirty-nine weeks and six days—a mere twenty-four hours short of my due date—when I dialed the physician who oversaw the prenatal program. He was a polite man whom I had met twice before (including a time when I had to tell him that his ultrasound technician used the wrong pronoun when referring to me). He didn't answer, but called me back an hour later.

"I went to a chiropractor and I have rib separation. I'm in so much pain. I can't sleep. The American Society of Obstetrics and Gynecology says that induction at thirty-eight weeks is fine if the baby is measuring at term and if the pregnant person is otherwise healthy and the pregnancy has been uneventful. My pregnancy *has been* uneventful. I've been your most boring patient. This baby is ready to be born. They're fully cooked. Please schedule me for an induction. *Please.*"

There was silence. Maybe it was the shock of listening to a pregnant man crying on the phone—at that point, I *was* crying—or maybe it was the fact that my due date was the next day, but when he finally spoke, he said, "I can call in the induction for tomorrow morning. Okay?" I couldn't control the sudden swift intake and slow exhale of my breath. The relief I felt came out as a giddy, still-crying sort of giggle.

"Oh my god. Really? Tomorrow?! Thank you. Thank you! What do I do? Do I call them? What time should I be there?" Biff and the kids overheard and started scrambling around the living room in excitement.

"He's being born tomorrow??!!!" Hailey shrieked and started running around the house in circles. I tried to shush her so I could hear the doctor.

"I have submitted the order into the system, and they'll call you tonight to schedule it. They've been pretty backed up over there so they may have to reschedule you, just so you know." I was relieved.

"Oh no they won't," I insisted. "I'm getting this baby out of me tomorrow. You'll see."

As I hung up the phone, I remembered that a photographer was in our living room. She had traveled to Portland to interview us for BuzzFeed and to capture the final moments of my pregnancy. I ushered everyone else outside, and she captured photos of Hailey's weeping, smiling face as she embraced me over and over again. And I cried, too, knowing that our lives were about to change again.

We made all our plans, packed the "go bag," and arranged for my parents to pick up the kids from Biff's parents the following day. My dad had wanted to be there for the birth, so once the induction time was set, he and my mom left Canada to head for Portland. Whether from pain or excitement or fear, I couldn't sleep that night. Instead, I focused on my breathing, slipping in and out of a meditative state in which I tried to connect with the spirit or the body of this little formative being. I tried to tell the baby that we were so excited to meet him, and that it would be a hard couple of days, but we were going to get through it together. I lay there with my hands on my belly all night, trying to manage the pain of my skin stretching beyond its ability and my ribs pulling in and out of their connective tissues, trying to manage the fear of labor and childbirth, trying to manage the excitement of finally meeting this human I had been growing inside of me. I hummed off and on throughout the night, the vibrations soothing my vagus nerve and, I hoped, carrying into the fetus's nervous system as well. They had been hearing my breaths, my heartbeat, the faint echo of my speaking and singing voice for as long as they had existed, from the very moment they transitioned from a cell to a cluster of cells, from when they were a blastocyst and then an embryo, from the creation of their brain and the final evolution of their ears and hearing system and the connection of that brain and those ears. My breath and my heartbeat and my voice, the wet sounds of their own hiccups and fetal movements—that had been their whole world, and all of that was about to change. The baby and I were about to work together, along with my medical team, to bring them into the outside world, which would be so very different than everything they'd ever known.

My quiet humming and reassuring self-whispers got me through the night (and Biff lovingly tolerated them, although

I'm sure he would have preferred a silent bed partner on the final night before becoming a parent to a newborn baby). The morning was a blur of energy and excitement. Biff captured a video of us in the car heading to drop the kids off at Mark and Kimberley's house. Even Lucas looks excited, too overcome by the possibility of new life to be nervous about how our family dynamic might change. In the car, I received a call from the head nurse at the hospital on the east side. She let me know that they were full that morning, and that she was rescheduling me for the following day instead. *Oh, hell no.* I rushed through possible responses, fixated on the desired result of having my baby as soon as possible. *What will she respond best to?* I asked myself. *Rage? Pity? Should I ask to speak to her manager?!* I chose pity, hoping to play on her emotions by letting my own bubble to the surface.

"I'm so sorry," I apologized for my obvious emotional response (though not for *having* feelings). "I just have rib separation and am in so much pain and I really, really need to give birth *today*. What other options can you help me think through?" My vulnerability must have inspired her empathy, because I could hear her scrambling for ideas.

"We can put you on a waiting list for later today?" she suggested, but the uncertainty of that scenario only made me cry harder. "Or!" she exclaimed. "I could call the west side location to see if they have room!"

I allowed my relief to swim through the phone lines and said, "Oh my gosh. Would you? I would be so, so appreciative. Thank you so much!" I gushed as I got off the phone. Biff shook his head in disbelief at my theatrics, certain that I was putting on a show for sympathy. "What?" I feigned innocence. "I *am* upset! I just let her see it! I am not having this baby tomorrow. I am having it *today.*"

As we dropped the kids off with Biff's parents, the phone rang again. The woman on the line introduced herself as the head nurse at the west side hospital's labor and delivery ward. "We're a brand-new hospital and have lots of room for you."

"Great!" I exclaimed, typing the address into Biff's phone map and gesturing to him to start driving. "Also, I have to let you know that I'm a man." I tried to sound as open and inoffensive as possible. I needed her to feel excited to welcome a man into her wing of the hospital, and to not feel that I would be defensive or mean. This attitude of self-confidence and positivity is one I have cultivated as a survival mechanism to help me through a transphobic world. It is not the right way to survive or the only way to survive—it's just *my* way of surviving, and it's worked in my life so far.

I could sense her nodding through the phone as she reassured me that they'd had a trans nurse on the ward in the past year, and that he had helped train them, so they were prepared. I added, "Since you're the head nurse, I'm going to put you in charge of making sure that whatever midwife you assign me, that they're going to be supportive. Can you do that?" She said she knew exactly who to give me. I also told her, "And I want everyone—the person who brings me food, the person who changes my trash—*everyone* to know exactly what to expect when they come into my room, okay? I just can't be dealing with transphobia or weird faces when I'm also trying to have a baby."

"I'm on it," she said as we got off the call. I breathed a sigh of relief and tilted my seat back, closing my eyes and controlling my breathing while Biff drove us to the new birthing location. I heard Biff say, "We're going to meet our baby today" as I drifted into a half sleep, listening to the clicking of the turn signal, the road rushing by us, and the podcast Biff put on the radio as a distraction. "We're going to meet our baby today."

SPOILER ALERT: WE DID NOT meet our baby that day. As it turns out, labor can either be supershort or superlong. Mine was superlong. The hospital staff were determined to oversee a slow, gentle induction process (while I, on the other hand, was ready to push that baby out as fast as possible). They wanted to introduce each induction step gradually, allowing plenty of time for my body to respond to the stimulus being presented to it. The staff was amazing at telling me ahead of time what they were going to do and allowing me to ask questions along the way. They always let me know what the alternatives to each procedure were and what would happen if we chose to do nothing. This is in alignment with trauma-informed care, a medical approach that understands the many ways in which patients (especially those who are LGBTQ and/or people of color) have been mistreated socially, culturally, medically, or even historically. Trauma-informed care teaches providers that mistreatment, when it rises to the point of causing trauma, manifests in many ways; it teaches providers how to share power and control with patients and it encourages them to ask permission before any procedure.

I was taught, by a doula friend, the **BRAIN** method of decision-making during labor, and I used it throughout the two days I was hospitalized prior to giving birth. When presented with a choice, such as whether to continue with the next induction procedure or not, I asked what the **B**enefits of that procedure were, what the **R**isks were, what the **A**lternatives to the procedure might be, listened to my **I**ntuition about what we should do next, and asked what would happen if we did **N**othing. I have complicated feelings about the concept of "intuition," but I still teach the **BRAIN** method to trans folks for use in non-delivery settings as well—it's a great way to remind yourself to be an empowered, take-charge patient.

Soon after I'd been admitted, after they had given me a medicine that they'd hoped might jump-start labor, the OB-GYN on duty stopped by. He shook my hand and sat down next to the bed so he would be eye to eye with me (rather than towering over me, which can emphasize the power dynamic between doctor and patient). I noticed this small gesture and appreciated it.

"Hopefully you never have to see me again," he said jovially. "If all goes as planned, you'll be solely in the excellent care of the nurse midwives here; they'll take great care of you. But should you need me, I'll be just a few feet away during your whole process."

"Thanks!" I responded. "But just so you know, I am not interested in avoiding a birth by cesarean. The second you think something is wrong, cut this baby out of me. I don't care how I give birth—I just want to leave this hospital alive and with a baby who is also alive. Preferably with both of us untraumatized. I don't care how that happens."

He chuckled, and I saw Biff rolling his eyes in my peripheral vision. "There's no reason to believe that we'll go that route. Let's just focus on things going as planned, and we will deal with any emergencies as they arise." He glanced at my chart before returning his gaze to me. "Oh, one thing I did want to mark as a preference here. If you do need a C-section, for your health or the health of the baby—and I'm not saying that will happen, but just in case—one option is for me to make a vertical incision, as opposed to a horizontal one. Do you have a preference there?"

I had never seen a vertical cesarean scar; I didn't know it was possible, nor did I know why it might be preferable. I must have looked confused, because he explained further.

"Some people might feel that a horizontal scar at the bathing suit line is indicative of a C-section, and those people might associate that type of scar with femininity. However," he continued, "many men have a vertical scar between their navel and their pubic bone, which could be the result of any number of abdominal surgeries. I was simply considering that a verti-cal scar might be more affirming of your gender, and the data shows that cesarean delivery and postpartum outcomes are identical, regardless of the type of incision you have."

I was truly shocked by this suggestion. I had never heard of a vertical cesarean incision and was blown away by this phy-sician's attention to my gender identity. He had clearly done a lot of thinking about how to creatively attend to the needs of trans people. This type of next-level allyship was so rare that I almost couldn't speak! When I finally regained my words, I told him that yes, I would like a vertical incision. He reassured me once again that we probably wouldn't even need to think about a C-section, but that he wanted to be prepared just in case. We shook hands again and he left.

PART OF ME was terrified to be induced, even though I had spent weeks asking for it. I had spent so much time online read-ing birth stories and posts in birthing groups, and the words from the naturopath I spoke to in my final trimester continued to haunt me long past the point at which I had realized that this person and I did not share the same goals or worldview: "Don't *let* them induce you." "Pitocin is poison." "Induced labors are harder than natural labors." The position of me as a powerless person was so clear in these statements, as was the judgment of hospitals, medical staff, and a medicalized birth.

Every part of the induction went exactly as it should have, and within twelve hours it was time for them to put me on

Pitocin to increase the frequency of my contractions. I knew I wanted this labor to progress but because of what I had been told, I was also scared of this next step. Then I remembered that those words were shared by the same person who told me to take castor oil—actually poisonous if misused—and I was able to relax. As with anxiety that hit during my pregnancy, I tried to make friends with this fear, to reason with it: *Thank you for reminding me to keep myself and this baby safe. I am listening. But also, it's time for you to go now.*

Though people say you forget the pain of childbirth after it happens, I don't think I inherited that gene. I remember very clearly how uncomfortable each contraction was, how much pain my ribs were in, how hard it was to breathe. They put a heating pad under my back, which made me so hot that the air conditioner had to be set to its coldest setting. I remember demanding that they turn the air conditioner up higher as my support team (Biff, Kimberley, and my dad) layered on more and more sweaters. Once the epidural kicked in, the nurse was able to remove the heating pad, and the room temperature returned to a more comfortable range. The anesthesia caused the searing pain from my ribs to subside, and I was able to feel with my fingers where my ribs were popping out along my sternum with each breath I took. It was unnerving but also comforting, in a way. Though my pain had been dismissed as "regular pregnancy pain," my experiences had *not* been "regular." It was nice to know that I hadn't been a weak man who couldn't handle the usual tortures of pregnancy. I had been a normal man who couldn't handle the particular torture of growing a baby that was too big for his body.

The epidural also meant that I was finally able to rest, midway through my labor. I hadn't been pain-free in weeks, and the relief was glorious. Having an epidural didn't prevent my body from producing the same chemicals that are normally produced during labor—I experienced the same high highs and low lows as everyone else. At one point, I felt my body flush with energy and joy. I felt as connected to the experience and those in the room as I have ever felt connected to anything. I called Biff over to me as tears streamed down my face, holding his hand and repeating, "We're going to meet our baby! We're going to meet our baby!" Ever the stoic, Biff simply raised his eyebrows and nodded his head. I continued, "There's no one else in the world I would rather be doing this with." It felt romantic and profound to say this aloud, but Biff burst into laughter and so did his mom.

"I should hope not!" he exclaimed, shaking his head at my sentimentality. I didn't care. I was overcome with bliss and rode the wave until I drifted off to sleep.

Then it was time to push. The nurse adjusted my bed and the lights, and I felt all the joy and energy and love seep from my body as if I had taken opioids. Even blinking my eyes felt like a Herculean task I was unprepared to do. My breaths became slow and heavy, my head a weight upon my shoulders. *This is what death feels like*, I remember thinking. *I am going to die.* I reached for Biff's hand and held it, weakly.

"I'm so sorry," I told him, slowly shaking my head. "I can't do this. I can't have our baby." My breath rattled in my chest as the machines around me whirred and beeped. I turned my head toward the nurse who was still adjusting the room's setup. I told her, "I'm going to die."

I hadn't meant to be dramatic; none of this was for any desired effect. I simply felt that these were my last moments on this earth. I had never felt so drained in my life. I had been unable to eat for the past 24 hours, throwing up even the Gatorade, water, and ice they had given me. Jell-O, lollipops— everything had come up mere minutes after being consumed. I had nothing left to give to this process and was ready to drift away to whatever comes after life.

The nurse had seen this before, of course. She crouched down so we were nearly nose to nose, and in her no-nonsense Super Nanny accent she told me, "I've been doing this for twenty years, and I haven't lost anyone yet. I promise you, you are not going to die." She was so adamant, so certain, her words stirred the beginnings of strength. Her voice lowered and she said to me, "You're doing a great job. The *best* job. No one on earth is doing as great a job as you are, right now." She nodded her head in agreement with herself, and I found myself nodding along with her. *She's right*, I thought. *I am doing the best job. I CAN do this. I can have this baby!*

I turned back to Biff and said, "Let's do this." Then I remembered that I didn't know what "this" even was. "Actually, I don't know what to do." I began to panic. "I don't know what to do!" I said to the nurse as she left the room to get the rest of the birthing team.

"Yes, you do!" she called over her shoulder. "We'll help you!"

AND SUDDENLY THE ROOM TRANSFORMS from a hospital room to a delivery room. My bed is flat, and my feet are in stirrups. Lights appear in the ceiling, pointed toward my crotch. I remind Biff that I don't want him to look down there except when the head is crowning; I am too afraid of what he might see, afraid it might break his attraction to me. Biff holds my left hand, and my dad holds my right. Biff's mother, Kimberley, stands beside him in support. Someone explains that when I feel the wave of a contraction come, I must push along with it to help things along. There is pain, and I close my eyes and count to five, imagining myself on my favorite bench on the cliffs of Orcas Island, the ocean in front of me, the forest behind me. A contraction comes, and I push and scream. Someone tells me not to yell—to put all of that yelling energy into the pushing. "But they do it in the movies!" I protest.

"That's not real!" the nurse retorts before telling me to push again.

She comes around from my feet to talk to me, saying that if I'm not able to push well enough, they can always take out the epidural so I can feel what I'm doing better. This gives me a renewed sense of urgency and I push as hard as I can, given that I can't feel what I'm doing. My dad and Kimberley and Biff and the nurses are all cheering me on. I try to remember the visualizations—I am a flower blooming, a door opening, a dam bursting. I am water rushing down a river, the ocean giving and taking, a drop of rain bursting as it hits the forest floor.

The next few times I push, I throw up all over myself and my support people. "I'm so sorry!" I try to exclaim, but everyone shushes me, reminding me to keep pushing as they wipe my face and shirt with warm, wet towels. Someone tells me to "use the energy of throwing up to push harder!" Someone else tells me I'm almost done, they can see the head. "You're just saying that to make me keep going!" I insist. Doubtfully, I give them a test. "What color is his hair?"

She says, "It's black!" I decide she's not lying after all and commit to pressing onward.

Then time slows down. I open my eyes and Biff and my dad are holding my hands, urging me to push. I close my eyes and my people, my ancestors, are in the room with me. The giving and taking of life stretch out in front of me, and I feel the presence of all the people I have come from, and all the people who will come from me. I open my eyes again and there are more presences in the room—I imagine that the ghost of my friend Annie, who officiated our wedding and passed away two years later, is in the room, too, telling me to find the joy in this powerful, sacred moment. I close my eyes and push, seeking the joy of this experience that is connecting me to the river of my family. I open my eyes and it's as if the ghost of my beloved teacher Patricia is there too, telling me to find the beauty in this visceral, painful moment. This child birthing experience that she never got to have, that she is so thrilled I am living through. I close my eyes and push, reveling in how beautiful it is to have lived this life where I get to be here, now, in this hospital with these people bringing this baby into the world. When I open my eyes, the room is full—Annie and Patricia and every other ghost I need to conjure to finish this epic process I began all those years ago when I first saw Biff across the street and knew that he was going to change my life forever.

I find Biff's eyes, and he squeezes my hand one last time as voices cry out over the din, telling me to stop pushing, to slow down, to breathe. Everything is still and silent for a split second, then there is a wet, slurping sound and I feel my body release. I look up and someone is holding my baby up and I see him against the bright lights, his black hair matted to his cone-shaped head, his red face squished up in surprise. He lets out a cry that echoes into my bones as if he is saying, "I am here!" The nurses rush to put a striped hat on his head and place him naked onto my bare chest. As soon as he feels my skin he stops crying and begins cooing—the softest, sweetest sound I've ever heard.

I am stunned by his beauty. I don't know what he will be like—what he *is* like—but I am overwhelmed by the deep, rushing waters of love. I move him just the slightest bit so I can see his face, to make sure he is ordinary. Yes, the fear of giving birth to a monster sneaks into this perfect moment too. And he is completely, wonderfully ordinary. But of course, to me, he is anything but ordinary in the sense of who and what he is. And I realize, in that moment, that whatever his body looked like when he came to us—I would always only see him as perfect. As more than perfect. As wonderful. As powerful. As mine. But also not mine—as himself. A little bit me, a little bit Biff, completely himself.

A nurse asks what we plan to name him, and I tell her, "Leo." Biff's middle name. Short and sweet and strong. Leo. He feels like a baby bird on my chest, and we lie there like that, skin to skin, for a long time. Eventually I give him to Biff, to share this golden time where things are simpler than they will ever be for the rest of our lives. When we are just loving humans, like every human throughout all of time, who have brought a new life into this world. Nothing more than that, and nothing less. Just humans.

Notes from Life in Our Family

Get Powerful.

If you're pregnant or plan to get pregnant, have you thought about what you need to feel safe, secure, and empowered during your birth? There are so many voices telling you to do this or that, and many of those opinions come from the opinion-giver's trauma or from a rigid understanding of what birth "should" or "shouldn't" be. For me, I was very sure about how I wanted my birth to go—in a hospital, with a doctor nearby. As it became clear that my body wasn't going to go into labor on its own, and as the fetus continued to grow larger and larger, straining my narrow frame, it also became clear that I wanted to be medically induced. But I kept doubting myself, going to different sources for comfort and assistance without understanding that each source would also have its own analysis of the world.

Because I am supernaturally optimistic, I'm going to assume that at no point did my midwife think, *How can I make Trystan's pregnancy more miserable?* And I'm also going to assume that at no point did the naturopath think, *How can I make Trystan put unknown substances into his body and shame him for his birth choices?* But damn, did those two extremes drive me into a shaking, fearful spiral. Pay attention to yourself; when you're in a fear spiral take a step back and find people who will help you access that part of yourself that feels powerful again.

Get Connected.

Whenever you want something that is different from what another person is trying to give you, just ask yourself: What is this person's motivation in this moment? Is it to work less, to serve people, to feel good about themselves, to not get sued? What do they care about most? Then connect to that motivation as you make your case. For me, building empathy and getting people excited about being on my "team" was how I managed to get an induction scheduled, how I avoided a postponed induction, and how I built a supportive team of birthing professionals at the hospital where I did give birth.

Get Endurance.

When you're pregnant or a new parent, everyone has opinions for you. Here are six tips to survive other people's opinions:

1. Maintain your privacy. It's okay to keep some things to yourself! You don't have to share every detail of your birth or parenting plan. If someone is being nosy, thank them for their interest and let them know you're keeping that information private.

2. Acknowledge their opinion, and let it go. I like the phrase "We will keep that in mind." It works for all kinds of situations to let someone know you've heard them and will consider it, but you're not interested in discussing it further.

3. Ask parents you respect for advice. If you notice that someone else's kids are well behaved or polite, don't be afraid to ask them for tips.

4. Look for logic. Remember that "intuition" can be influenced by many factors, including personal bias and past trauma. Ask yourself: Is there evidence to support your decision?

5. Don't be afraid to change your mind. Whether it's related to your birthing or feeding plan, your pregnancy experience or parenting in general, it's okay to realize your idea didn't match reality and to adjust accordingly. Try to hold lightly to all of your plans.

6. If you have a partner (or partners), lean on them. If someone does give you advice and you're not sure if it would make sense in your situation, check in with your partner! Chances are they will balance out your ideology and help you find middle ground.

CHAPTER NINE

HOW WE DO PARENTING

⌣

"Why have you chosen to assign a gender to your child?"

This was a question I was prepared to hear, but not entirely prepared to answer. The reason I told my story publicly was to make the world a better place for trans people, and I feel accountable to the community. If they aren't happy with what I'm doing, then I have failed.

Of course, I understand that the trans community isn't a monolith, and that many of us are so traumatized by a transphobic world that we are unable to navigate it in healthy ways. I know that there are some trans people who will never be happy with what they see me doing, because the world has been so harsh toward them that everyone's actions are viewed through a lens of trauma. I know that. But criticism from other trans people still stings more than that from non-trans people. I have such a deep and abiding love for them that—even when they are being unfairly critical—I take their every comment to heart.

When I posted the first public photo of newborn Leo and saw that the very first comment on the photo was from a trans person admonishing us for assigning a gender to our baby, my heart broke. In truth, I was angry at this person. *Who looks at a picture of a newborn baby and, instead of appreciating the new life that another trans person has created, decides to criticize that trans person who went through hell to have this baby?! Who does that? And who doesn't have the empathy and love and compassion that it takes to hit pause on their reaction for a split second to consider how that reaction might impact the trans person who made themselves vulnerable to the whole world?*

Unfortunately, I hadn't yet learned the skill of letting myself have that reaction quietly. Now, three years later, I have made friends with this reaction and am practiced at pausing and working through it internally. I have a whole system where I remind myself that a stranger on the internet doesn't have the power to hurt me. That the person posting the comment has their own very real experiences of harm around gender. That the harm they've experienced is causing them to lash out at me. I remind myself that it is transphobia that I am mad at, since it is transphobia that has hurt this person in this way. In fact, this person

HOW WE DO PARENTING

and I are *both* mad at transphobia, so if I can convince them to join me, we can *both* fight transphobia instead of each other.

But alas, I had not learned those skills just after Leo was born, and so I reacted to this person . . . right in the comments section, badly. I went off on them for having the audacity to comment on a newborn baby photo with a judgmental message. Luckily, Biff saw the whole thing just a few hours later and deleted the comment and my response to it, reminding me that I was supposed to stay away from comments entirely. He was right, of course, and over the next few months I developed healthy ways to explain our approach to gender for anyone who is curious.

I was not angry that someone was asking why we called Leo "he" when he was born, or why we gave him a traditionally male name. I was angry that people assumed we just defaulted to the cultural norm without thinking about it. Of course we thought about it—we're queer! I'm transgender! In many ways, I feel like I've gone through the looking glass of gender and am viewing it from the other side. Neither Biff nor I believe that simply picking a pronoun for your child is inherently harmful. Others disagree, which is okay! It should go without saying that many trans people disagree with each other on a whole host of topics. But Biff and I believed that Leo was just as likely to feel unsettled by a gender-neutral name and/or pronoun. I often joke that Leo was "diagnosed male." There is no neutrality with gender, no complete absence of gender.

A "gender-neutral" name is still a name, and gender-neutral pronouns are still pronouns. Giving your child any name or assigning pronouns is still a choice that you are making on behalf of your child—one that they are just as likely to feel harmed by as a name or pronoun typically associated with masculinity or femininity.

For us, it was a numbers game. Leo is most likely to feel comfortable being referred to as a boy, compared to the other options available. So we chose to call him a boy and to use he/him pronouns until and unless he tells us he wants to go by something else. Did I love it when strangers called him "a strong little man" and insinuated that he was "flirting" with girls, even before he could talk? No. But I also couldn't bear the burden of educating every fool person I met at the grocery store. We had done so much for so long, inviting strangers and cameras into our lives for the entire pregnancy process, that we needed a break.

WHEN LEO WAS BORN, we were intentional about not making assumptions about who would do what. We discussed every aspect of how we wanted to raise a baby together and came to the decision that I would not be bodyfeeding Leo.* Even though I felt 100 percent certain that this was the right decision for

---

*A note about terminology: I use "breastfeeding," "chestfeeding," "nursing," and "bodyfeeding" interchangeably. There is currently no universal word or term to describe the act of feeding one's baby using one's body, so I'm just going to use them all.

us, so too did I feel certain about keeping the decision private. In fact, this was one of three things that my mother urged me to keep to myself.

"I don't like to give advice," she said when I was just a few months pregnant. "But . . . sometimes it's best to not tell people what you plan to name your baby, until the name is already on the birth certificate. I also recommend not sharing how you plan to feed the baby, because people have all kinds of stupid opinions about that. And finally, it's best not to share how you plan to give birth, because inevitably people will tell you their horror stories, and you don't need that going into your labor."

It was good advice, and I took it. Hundreds of strangers on the internet asked me if I was going to breastfeed; so did journalists live on TV; so did every medical professional I encountered at every prenatal checkup I attended. I wanted to scream it from the mountaintops: STOP ASKING ABOUT MY BREASTS!!! But of course, I couldn't do that. Other than my medical team, I told everyone the same thing: "Thanks for your concern, but we aren't sharing that information publicly."

Every trans person has to be extremely careful when talking about our bodies. We have seen celebrities expertly navigate this invasive curiosity in the media, and when it comes to explaining why this obsession is so troubling, they've done a better job than I ever will. What I can say is that I knew, from my years of experience working with the media, that I couldn't talk about my genitalia, my sex life, or my breasts without sending the vast majority of the audience down a dark trail of transphobic thoughts. It's just a psychological trigger for people who are on the fence or who don't know a lot about trans people. Transphobia, much like racism, is a complicated series of psychological tripwires. To truly uproot any bias, one must be a ninja of sorts, dancing around and dodging the common stereotypes that can send someone reeling backward, away from acceptance. So I kept it to myself, and I'm glad that I did.

Now that it's in the past, I feel comfortable talking about why we chose to formula feed. Part of the decision was simple: I just didn't resonate with the cultural obsession with breastfeeding. There are huge subsets of the internet filled with hot takes on bottle- and formula-feeding parents. There are hundreds of memes about how formula feeding parents are "lazy" or just don't love their children enough . . . or at all.

I didn't even *tell* people that we were planning to use formula and I was *still* subjected to emails and comments about how my baby would grow up sickly if I used formula.

The other truth is: *I just didn't want to chestfeed.* I didn't want to use my body in that way. I wasn't comfortable with it. And I wanted to make sure that Biff and Leo got some precious newborn bonding time, that I didn't hoard the biological connection I had with Leo. After all, my body had nourished his body for nine months! Watching Biff (and Hailey and my parents and Biff's parents) feed Leo in those first few weeks of his life are some of my sweetest memories. I'm grateful that I was able to share that nurturing experience with my family members, so they could all experience what it is like to nourish a tiny human. I was also grateful for the ability to care for myself by sleeping at night while Biff got up to do feedings. Healing from pregnancy and labor proved more difficult than I thought it would be, and having the ability to focus on my fourth-trimester body was a gift.

I also wanted to give as much love and attention to Lucas and Hailey as possible; I felt that those initial weeks as a family of five would be crucial as a blueprint for our future. Both children, whom we quickly nicknamed "the big kids," had been tender and emotional upon meeting Leo for the first time. They jostled their way into the hospital room just a few minutes after the nurses had everything cleaned up, and they each got to hold all nine pounds of him (I told you he was a big baby!). In the postpartum period I tried to take them to the park or the museum, leaving Leo home with Biff or Kimberley, so they would know that I was still their dad, even in this new family formation. Hailey spent hours singing to Leo, playing peekaboo, picking out outfits for him, and squealing about his funny faces or poopy diaper. I still read her bedtime stories and tried to do my usual neighborhood walks with Lucas as well.

I could only do so much, though, because I found it physically difficult to be away from Leo for too long. The strength of my connection to him was surprising and a bit unnerving. Friends had warned me about postpartum anxiety, depression, and the like, but no one had mentioned that I might experience the opposite, a kind of postpartum elation. I wanted to be holding him as often as possible, for hours at a time, preferably. There was a kind of spiritual umbilical cord that had not been cut, and I felt deeply aware of his every experience. A slightly furrowed brow or a clench of a tiny hand told me all I needed to know: "He's hungry," I would declare. "He's cold." Being his dad was the only thing I've ever been perfect at, and it required no effort at all.

When it comes to trans fertility, there are three things that keep me up at night. One is the fertility of transgender women, about which almost no research has been done. Two is the fertility of transgender youth, who are making lifesaving decisions that may impede their ability to ever be biological parents. And three is postpartum issues. Very little is known about the experiences of trans people postpartum, but anecdotally, I see a lot of perinatal mood disorders in my community. I am profoundly blessed to say I didn't experience mental health challenges as I was navigating life as a parent to a newborn, but I cannot wait until more is known about how and why some trans parents experience challenges while others thrive.

And boy, did I thrive. I expected parenting a newborn to be nearly impossible! But after the crash course in parenting Hailey and Lucas, a baby was easy. I got to do things I wish I'd done with the big kids when they were little, like really start to integrate the principles of consent from the beginning. If a child learns, from a very early age, that they have every right to say no to any kind of unwelcome touch, they are less likely to put up with any violation of their personal boundaries later on. With Leo, I practiced this by simply telling him that I was going to change his diaper before I did it. Easy, simple. Sometimes I would even ask him if it was okay for me to change his diaper at that moment. I knew he was not going to respond, but I wanted to get into the habit of asking permission to touch him before I actually did it.

My friend Stephen, who was a nanny for many years, also told me that it is helpful to narrate when you are changing a baby's diaper, because it lays the groundwork for future potty training. So, telling Leo what I was going to do served both the purpose of getting his consent *and* engaging him in the diaper-changing process. By the time Leo was two months old, he was lifting up his own bottom to "help" me change his diaper, and by the time he was six months old, he was telling us when he needed a diaper change.

As he became a toddler, Leo also loved to play "the tickle game," which is a game where he would tell me to tickle him and I did, and then he would tell me to stop and I stopped. That's it. That's the whole game. It allowed him to practice saying yes and no, and having his yes and no be respected.

WE WERE ALSO ABLE to really commit to gender-creative parenting in ways that we couldn't with Hailey and Lucas (because we were so worried about our actions being portrayed badly in court). We don't personally believe that harm is caused by simply assigning a gender to a child, but we do believe harm is caused by allowing gender to dictate too many aspects of childhood. Ever since Leo was born, we dressed him in outfits from across the gender spectrum. We grew his hair out when it was thick enough to look decent, and when he was old enough to express a desire to have it short again, we took him to get it cut. He loves his car toys and his baby doll that eats fake food. By age three he started to show a preference for clothing styles and often chooses clothes from the "girls" section.

Once, when I was looking at kids' clothes online in preparation for this third birthday, I pulled up the "boys" section by default and asked him to pick out an outfit. He nixed every single one. Realizing that my own gender bias was showing itself, I clicked over to the "girls" section, and his face lit up. He picked out several outfits that one might call *very* feminine (as in pink-striped ruffle-sleeved shirts with purses screen printed onto them). I bought them without making any mention of their intended gender, and he happily wears them everywhere we go. He still insists that he's a boy (actually, he says, "I a BIG BOY!"), but he has no way of knowing that the clothes he loves are traditionally found on girls. We are allowing him to explore gender however he wants, free from the judgment and constraints of our culture's rigid norms.

Because here's the thing—whether it's men learning how not to be sexist or it's white people learning how not to be racist, empathy is perhaps the most powerful tool of allyship. If Leo does go on to become a boy and then a man, it will only ever be a good thing that he embraced femininity at an early age. When men are at peace with the feminine aspects of themselves, they are not challenged by femininity in the world. When men don't see femininity as weak, they will not take advantage of feminine people. The cultures that punish femininity have more violence against women across the board—fear of women breeds violence toward women, and one way to reduce fear is to embrace femininity.

I have yet to meet a grown man who was upset that his parents allowed him to freely explore all the parts of himself when he was young. On the contrary, I have met many men who are scarred by parents who used force, shame, and coercion to enact rigid norms of masculinity upon them. When I work with high schoolers, I ask the boys to tell me when they've been ordered to "act like a man" or to "stop being a sissy." They always have dozens of examples, including—most shockingly—a young man who told the class about the time he was punished for crying after breaking his leg on the football field. Let that sink in: His dad and coach punished him for expressing emotion when he *broke his leg*. To me and Biff, *that's* the most harmful aspect of how we approach gender in our culture. *That's* the type of behavior that needs to shift if we ever hope to have a world in which one's gender doesn't imply anything about their strength, emotional capacity, or competence. Or heck, even a world where women and feminine people are seen as equal to men and masculine people.

In ways large and small, that's all I have ever wanted—and what I continue to fight for.

Whether it's telling our family's story or teaching Lucas that it's okay to cry, I am rebuilding the world around me with love. In this new empire, our family is protected from bias—and everyone is invited to join us. It is possible to take the broken shards of glass you've been given and craft a mosaic from the pieces—something more beautiful than what was there before.

Notes from Life in Our Family

Get Safe.

Do you have experiences of feeling unsafe, either as a kid or as a grown-up?

One way you can find healing around these memories is to empower your kids to avoid situations like the one you encountered, and to ensure that they won't grow up to be the type of person who can't respect boundaries. Don't be afraid to have those conversations with them in an age-appropriate way. Ask them questions about their experiences and remind them that no one should ever touch them in a way that they don't like. Practice with them so they know, in their bodies, how to respond if they are rejected or targeted. That way, if the time ever comes, they'll know what to do. And if they are unable to avoid a victimization situation, they'll feel safe enough to come to you as soon as possible.

EPILOGUE

UP UNTIL THE COVID-19 PANDEMIC, I traveled a lot for
work. And don't get me wrong—I love traveling. I love being
with people in other cities, seeing how they live. I love standing in front of a room: teaching doulas about trans inclusion,
teaching doctors about trauma-informed care, teaching com-
panies about equity and inclusion. I love airports and hotels
and hole-in-the-wall restaurants in New York's Little Italy or
Detroit's Food Truck Alley. But I don't love the fact that travel
takes me away from my family. I miss being with Biff and the
kids and feel guilty for jet-setting all over while he stays home
and keeps everything running. So, in 2018, I started bringing
a kid with me whenever I could afford it. I alternated which
kid I brought (one time Hailey, one time Lucas, and so on) so
that I could have critical one-on-one time with each of them in
different cities around the country. Lucas has been to Oakland
and San Francisco with me, Hailey to Los Angeles and San
Diego. Lucas was supposed to hit Chicago with me this year
(and Hailey and I were scheduled to do a three-city Texas tour)
but all of that was canceled when the pandemic hit.

It was the summer of 2019 when I took Hailey to LA and realized how important that long-term one-on-one time truly is. We were sitting in our rental car in LA traffic when Hailey, completely out of the blue, asked if anyone had ever said anything mean to me when I was pregnant. I paused, considering how I should answer this question—how much I should share with her.

"Yes," I finally said. "People did say mean things." Now it was her turn to pause, perhaps weighing whether and how to ask the next question she had on her mind.

"Well, I guess I'm wondering if you will tell me . . . what they said," she asked tentatively. "Like, what kinds of mean things did they tell you?"

I sighed, knowing that it would be a long time before I felt she was truly ready to hear the kinds of hateful, disgusting things I was subjected to while I was pregnant. Hailey has always believed herself to be supremely mature, ready for all information about everything, no matter how dark or disturbing. Of course, she believes this about herself because we have protected her from the worst elements of the world. I knew she would be disappointed, but I had to let her down. I tried to do it gently.

"Hm. You know, sweetheart, that's not something I'm going to share with you right now." She started to protest but I was firm. "You know one of my most important jobs is to protect your powerful spirit, and I think hearing those words would harm you in a way that might be impossible to fix."

She nodded, perhaps not understanding my reasoning but accepting my no as final. She was still curious, though, and pressed on.

"Did those things they said hurt your feelings?" She was already on the verge of empathic tears, I could tell. Her eyes were wide and wet.

"Yes," I admitted delicately. "They did, especially at first. But I had friends who helped keep the worst things away from me. And I worked to get strong in the ways I needed to be to survive. But yes, it hurt. And it still does sometimes."

"Did you ever cry?" she asked, a single tear sliding down her cheek. And though I knew it hurt her deeply to imagine her dad in pain, I truthfully nodded yes. The single tear was joined by two thin streams sliding down her rosy cheeks. I wondered where these questions were coming from—what she was truly asking. I felt that we were in a magical moment of connection and openness, so I asked a question I had been sitting with for a long time. I knew I would get an honest answer from her because of the energy of the moment.

"Do you ever wish you were in a different family? A more normal one?" I asked it as neutrally as I could so she would know that I wanted an honest answer, one that wasn't fabricated to protect me. But she was shaking her head before I was even done with the sentence.

"No!" she exclaimed, her eyes wide. "Never in a million, gajillion years." We both laughed at her hyperbole, and I told her that "million, gajillion" isn't a real number. But as the traffic eased and I returned my eyes to the road, I felt her hand on mine and smiled. Because actually, "a gajillion" might be the exact right way to think about our family. Not in a gajillion years has there been a family like us, nor will there be in another gajillion. And that's true for every family that has ever been. Each is exquisitely unique and painstakingly ordinary. Just like ours.

APPENDIX:
HOW WE DO ACTIVISM

AS PARENTS, BIFF AND I teach by example. Putting a lens up to our lived experiences as queer people, our lifelong commitment to anti-racism, and our inherited beliefs around justice, here are some lessons we've learned that you might find helpful.

Get Pro-Trans: Talking Trans with your Kids

"But how can a man have a baby?"

"Where's your mom? Is she dead?"

"I talked to my dad, and he said you're a liar. Only mommies can get pregnant."

Even in Portland, our liberal mecca (of sorts), I overhear kids saying outright nasty or just plain ignorant things to my kids. And yes, kids say the darnedest things. Even if they have parents who are loving and supportive and open, kids are still learning and growing and on their own little journeys. But I can't help but think: If more parents were talking about transgender people, my kids wouldn't have to do so much defending of themselves and educating of others. They could spend more time playing, learning, connecting, and having fun.

So how do you do that? Simple! Talk to your kids about transgender people! If you know someone who is trans, talk to your kid about them. If you don't know anyone who is trans, buy books about trans people and add them to your kids' shelves. Watch shows about trans people. Bring up trans issues with your family. It is never too early for kids to learn that there are all kinds of people with all kinds of gender identities and all kinds of bodies.

When Leo was two, we were sent a book that had a pregnant picture of me in it. Needless to say, Leo loves that book. Whenever we get to the page with me on it, he laughs with glee. "It's Daddy in my dook!" he exclaims. "And I in dook too—in Daddy's tummy!" He is never traumatized and never has any follow-up questions.

Kids are open and accepting, and the earlier you introduce ideas of difference to them, the easier it will be for them to move through those stages of learning and the less work you'll have to do apologizing for them when they're older.

You don't want to have to apologize for them. I've been on the receiving end of *many* apologies (on the playground, over email, walking down the street, picking up the kids from school) and it's super embarrassing for everyone involved. I would much rather that you show your kid my Instagram feed and talk to them about men having babies than have to elicit an apology after your kid has said something mean to my kid on the playground.

Kids are often so up on trans information and lingo that your little ones are bound to surpass you before too long. It's important to stay up-to-date, too! Practice using a gender-neutral pronoun, because they're not going anywhere (see what I did there?). Learn the newest ways that people are describing their genders, because language will continue to evolve. In the internet era, everyone is connected to each other and communities are working together to choose innovative ways of talking about themselves. Embrace humility as you learn and grow. Get excited to do better and be better in the world.

Does your family support trans rights? How would others know? Make sure you're working to take action in support of trans people on a regular basis. Whether it's advocating for a gender-neutral bathroom at your kids' school or speaking up at a city council meeting on nondiscrimination, practice telling your own trans ally story so others can follow in your footsteps!

Like, comment on, and share social media posts by trans organizers, artists, storytellers, and activists. High engagement with our followers translates to more college speaking gigs, more viewers for our ideas (which means more change in the world), and a better chance at selling a book (Heeeey!).

Listen to the stories you hear from trans people. Believe them. Take action when they tell you to. It's often not complicated to be a good ally—just pay attention when people tell you what they need!

Get Anti-Racist.

With the rising of a more universal awareness of systemic racism, I'm bombarded with messages about "how to be an anti-racist." In my professional life as a consultant, I'm often called upon to teach anti-racism. The first thing I'll say is, pay attention to Black voices.

If you're a white person, chances are that white supremacy lives somewhere in your heart, even after years of knowing it is wrong. Racism and anti-Blackness is the smog we've all been breathing in, our whole lives.

Anti-racism is the act of finding those artifacts of racist thought and action, bringing them into the light, and letting them go. It is showing up for your kids by talking openly about race and power and privilege, even if you don't have all the answers. It is being honest about your experiences and fears and doubts. And it's about taking action. As John Lewis suggested: Take action that is in alignment with your values (that's the hands). Do justice. Learn more, feel more, and act more.

My professional training in anti-racism is from four different schools of thought, and when I do anti-racism work, I pull from all of them. In the context of parenting, the most useful approach is the Developmental Model of Intercultural Sensitivity (a ridiculously long name for an extremely helpful tool). The DMIS is an evidence-based approach to understanding the different stages that people go through on their road to anti-racism. The theory is that there is nothing wrong with anyone's journey—every step along the way is critical to your final arrival at an anti-racist identity. This is particularly useful when approaching our children. Instead of judging where they are, we can calculate what stage they've reached and think strategically about how to move them forward.

The Developmental Model of Intercultural Sensitivity

I use this tool all the time when talking with my kids about race, gender, LGBTQ issues, disability, neurodiversity, and more. It helps me to stay connected and present with them as they ask questions, rather than snap to judgment or shame.

Stage One: **Denial.** In this stage, people don't pay particular attention to differences in culture. Some adults are still in this stage, but most children grow out of it quickly, especially if they live in a diverse neighborhood or are exposed to diversity in books and shows. Up until Leo was three or so, he was in this stage. He would point at Black girls in his books and tell me, "That look like you, Daddy!" The great news is that you don't need to do much to move kids out of this stage—just expose them to families that look different from yours and they'll move right along.

Stage Two: **Defense.** In this stage, people do notice difference and they perceive it as a threat. Our brains do this without us even trying! Most of the time humans have been alive, we've been under siege. Warring bands of people, tribes from other villages, plagues, lions, colonizers—you name it, humans have survived it. And the people who survived those threats were the most anxious, neurotic of the bunch. They stayed alive and gave birth to an even more anxious, neurotic next generation, and so on until eventually, you were born. And, if you're a parent, you gave birth or adopted kids who likely inherited the same aversion to difference that saved your ancestors from being slaughtered or eaten. It's natural to notice difference and it's even natural to be curious about it or defensive toward it. When kids point out differences in others' skin tones, body types, or family makeup, you may feel embarrassed or even ashamed, as if you've failed somehow. Good news! You haven't! But what you do next *matters*. Gently encourage your child to see that difference as good. "Yes, that person does have dark skin! Isn't it beautiful? It's so good to have people of all skin colors around us!" "Yes, that person does use a wheelchair to get around! Good noticing! Isn't it awesome that we all move differently?" And so on.

Stage Three: **Minimization.** This is where many people get stuck. They believe that difference can't really be a threat if it isn't that different at all. Kids in this stage will admonish you for pointing out difference and will tell you that we're "all the same inside." Often my anti-racism coaching clients will roll their eyes as they tell me about their parents' backward approach to race. "They told me they didn't see race! As if that was the goal!" I have to remind them that actually, this colorblind approach was pretty radical in the 1970s and '80s, and that their parents were just caught up in a national approach to difference at the time, when the goal *was* to better understand the similarities between groups of people, rather than the differences. It was an improvement over the Defense stage of the '50s and '60s, but still not the ideal resting place. When kids are at this stage, it's important to introduce them to ways that people who are different from them—which might be people of color if you're white and might be LGBTQ people if you're not LGBTQ—experience hardships they don't experience. I do this using the Socratic method, by asking them open-ended questions about the kids in their class or in their favorite shows, rather than by lecturing them. "So, I notice that the Black kid in this show doesn't have as many lines as the white kids. What's up with that?" Or "I don't see any families with two dads in these books. Why do you think that might be?"

Stage Three (My Addition): **Retreat.** Not everyone goes through this stage. For some, when going through these stages, they fall into retreat (especially if they're teenagers). When someone has been exposed to too much information about whiteness, white privilege, straight privilege, racism, anti-Blackness, sexism, transphobia, and so on, without an appropriate lens through which to process the information they've received, they fall into this stage: Overwhelmed by the knowledge of oppression, they turn inward and back away from further conversation or engagement around equality and justice. They may become depressed and wonder how they can continue, given the enormity of the task ahead of them. "If racism has always existed, how can I possibly make a difference?" "If white people are the problem and I'm white, I guess I don't have a role in this movement." I see a lot of despair in this stage, and the antidote is hope. If you're supporting someone who is in retreat, share hopeful messages about ways in which the world has changed and is still changing. As Mr. Rogers says, "Look for the helpers." If possible, support your young person in disconnecting from social media and the news for a while. Encourage them to pay attention to what is motivating them toward action against white supremacy, and what is contributing to a feeling of despair. Remind them that oppression feeds on despair and is starved by hope.

Stage Four: **Acceptance.** At this point, people realize that yes, there are people who are different than they are and yes, those differences matter. They are tacitly accepting of those differences, even if they might have judgments about them. To help your kids with acceptance, encourage them to learn about other cultures through exposure to media created by different voices, to other parts of the country and world, and to other cultures' stories.

Stage Five: **Adaptation.** People in this stage can both accept cultural differences and even adjust to fit in—"code switching" is not about performing a stereotype of that culture, but subtly (or even overtly) adjusting their mannerisms and communication style to better fit in with others. People in this stage are able to view the world through the eyes of another group and can understand (without being told) what language or mannerisms might be considered offensive or off-putting. The goal of allyship is adaptation: the ability to view the world through multiple lenses. For example, men who are in this stage will check how loud they are when speaking with women and are mindful of "mansplaining" or talking over women. White people in this stage are able to easily avoid even the most subtlety racialized language. Cisgender people in this stage know not to ask transgender people about their bodies or surgeries. Adaptation is the stage where your kids feel as comfortable around people who are different from them as they do when they're around those who are the same.

The Five-Step Intervention

The five-step intervention is a tool I've developed. I've used this with my parents, coworkers, strangers at the grocery store—pretty much anyone I come in contact with who engages in behavior that I think might be biased.

Before getting to the steps, let's start with a scenario. Here's what this might look like in practice:

Lucas storms into the kitchen where I am making a pot of tea. "Dada called me racist!" he declares. "This is outrageous!"

I turn around in a slow, silly way, drawing my eyebrows together as if I am a very serious old wise man in a movie. "Oh, really?" I say in a deep voice. "I am intrigued. Tell me more about what exactly you said. My office is open."

"I just said that I hate it that sometimes, the Black kids at my school bully nice white kids! How is that racist?" Lucas is fuming, as he often gets when he feels unfairly attacked. He is not able to let even the smallest critical comment go. I could understand why Lucas would be confused about this statement, since it wasn't inherently racist (per se). But I could also see why Biff perceived that Lucas may be making a broad generalization about *all* Black kids, missing the fact that Lucas might be universalizing his observations of one or two kids and also failing to recognize why kids of color might be seen as more rowdy or rambunctious than white kids. I was thrilled to have this conversation with Lucas, and I worked my way through my trusty steps:

1. Ask a question. Asking a question helps cut off your fight-or-flight response to a confrontation; it tells an anxious brain and body that this is just a conversation, and you are unlikely to get hurt here. It also reminds you that you are speaking to a human who is also on a journey—not a student you are about to lecture. When talking to Lucas I might ask, "Tell me a little bit more about when you see this happen at school. How does it make you feel?" Asking a question keeps your heart rate

down so you can stay calm. Kids sense anxiety like it's their superpower.

2. **Find commonality.** Finding commonality also helps you stay connected to the other person in the conversation, rather than going into lecture or shaming mode. With Lucas, I might say, "It sounds like when you see anyone being hurt, it reminds you of being hurt. Is that right? I hate seeing anyone get bullied. I understand why you would notice that." Relating to his perspective helps us both hold the space as sacred, and it cuts off his fight-or-flight response.

3. **Share impact.** As adults, or as people who have been doing the work of anti-racism for any amount of time at all, it's easy for us to view the world through the lens of the community being talked about. But for kids or others who haven't yet begun to sharpen the lens of allyship, the invitation to imagine their actions from the perspective of someone else will be a revelation. It will keep them out of their intention ("I didn't mean to be racist!") and will root them in impact (here's how someone might *hear* that as racist). I would say: "I wonder what it might feel like to you if you were Black, and you heard a white kid say that Black kids are bullies. How might that make you feel?" I'm building Lucas's empathy without him even knowing it.

4. Educate. With kids, I like to point out the wild tricks our brains can play on us. It depersonalizes the situation and helps keep things light, which is critical as we build up their confidence around issues of allyship. If shame creeps into the situation, we've already failed. As Brené Brown says, "Shame is the antithesis of social justice." Shame kills empathy, which is at the core of all allyship. This part also applies to adults; we can let kids know the history of the racist word they used without calling them a racist. Name-calling is a shame tactic, because it summarizes someone's entire being into a negative word rather than separating out who they are from what they've done. And once shame is in the mix, there is no way that your intervention will be effective. In practice, this might sound like: "One thing that our brains do is make connections even when there aren't any. For example, are there white kids who bully other white kids? Sometimes if one person of color does something, our brains tell us that *all* people of color do that thing. Isn't that silly?"

5. Appreciate. Closing on a positive note cements the learning, and if you're able to get someone to verbally commit to using different language or taking a different action in the future, that's even better. You might say, "Hey—it's okay to notice things, and I'm so glad you came to me. You can always talk to me. I'll never get mad at you, and I'm so proud you're able to listen and are open to learning." This is the science of change.

These steps are not hard! We know how brains work! We know where bias comes from, and we know how to create the most effective structures to help us uproot it. But it does require time and effort, and you may not have the time to do all five steps every time you notice racism. This method may not work for everyone or every situation, but when it comes to your kids, it's worth it to try—and you will raise a good human.

Whichever model you use, try to view your child/ren as people you're walking with, not pushing or pulling in any one direction.

Get Equality.

What are your kids passionate about? Whether it's animals or nature or playgrounds or almost anything—you can find a way to use that passion to ignite a fire of justice within your child. Start small, encouraging them to see what barriers might exist for their passion to fully thrive in our current climate. Are there any homeless animals in your area? Who is caring for them? Do they need volunteers or state funds? Is your city working to build a new playground in an area that doesn't have one?

Work with your family to build their empathy—ask your kids if they can imagine being an animal without a loving home, a kid without a playground, a deer without a forest. Gently support them to take action to make the world a better place, using whatever they're already excited about.

For example, Lucas is obsessed with YouTube, so I pitched an idea to him for a YouTube series encouraging kids to go on hiking trips with their parents. He loved it, and we ended up spending an entire day outside in the woods making videos. I also suggested that he research the names and stories of the indigenous people who stewarded the land long before anyone else got there, and he ended up deep in the Clackamas's history before he discovered that we have several friends who are Clackamas people! He gives a special acknowledgment at the beginning of his video, honoring their commitment to the beautiful land we were hiking on.

If allyship is the ability to see the world using multiple lenses, it's never too early to start honing your lens, and your kids' lenses, and your community's lens. When there is injustice, no matter how small, help your children see it. When it is right for them to take action, support them in doing so. And when they want to stage a walkout with protest signs at their middle school . . . for god's sake, buy them the paints.

ACKNOWLEDGMENTS

Trystan and his husband, Biff, live together with their three children, Lucas, Hailey, and Leo, on the unceded traditional homelands of the Clackamas band of the Chinook, the Watlala band of the Chinook, Cowlitz, Kathlamet, Multnomah, the Willamette Tumwater, the Wasco-Wishram, the Atfalati band of the Kalapuya, and the Tualatin Kalapuya, in what is now known as Portland, Oregon.

The events described in this book occurred on the unceded Indigenous lands of the Clackamas, Cascades, and Cowlitz people, or what is now known as Portland, Oregon.

We honor the Indigenous people whose traditional and ancestral homelands this book was written on: the Multnomah, Kathlamet, Clackamas, Tumwater, Watlala bands of the Chinook, the Tualatin Kalapuya, and many other Indigenous Nations of the Columbia River. It is important to acknowledge the ancestors of this place and to recognize that we are here because of the sacrifices forced upon them. In remembering these communities, we honor their legacy, their lives, and their descendants.

FIRST AND FOREMOST, I have the deepest appreciation for Biff, who held it down at home while I secreted away to various locations without Wi-Fi or cell service so I could write and not get distracted.

My agent, Myrsini Stephanides, for emailing me out of the blue and convincing me that, somehow, I could write a book.

My publisher, The Experiment, for taking a chance on a not-at-all-famous trans guy who wanted to write a not-quite-memoir about parenting.

My editor, Batya Rosenblum, for her tireless attention to detail, unapologetic streamlining, and candid feedback. Without you, this book would easily be half as good as it is!

Joshua Lyons, for his incredibly focused, caring attention and writing support as we crafted that very first pitch. And for modeling the solid no that led me to write the damn thing myself.

Thank you to my dear friend Wade McCollum, who encouraged me to start making notes along the way, in case I ever wrote a book one day.

Robin Stevenson, for teaching me how to organize my time, how to get unstuck, and how to believe that I had a story worth sharing.

Andrew Solomon, for his enthusiasm and support, and super practical help on marketing and PR.

My friends, Ryan and Sacha Luria, for saying yes when I wasn't sure how to make this happen, and for wanting a trans parenting book so badly that you were willing to be my first investors.

My mother, Janet, who said, "It's your story to tell and you can't hurt my feelings" when I asked if she wanted to read any of it. The next book might be about you—about us—and then you'll *have* to read it in advance.

My father, Clay, who has always shown me (and the world) more patience and love than any of us deserve.

My in-laws, Kimberley and Mark, who have allowed me to share parts of their story in these pages.

My sisters, Sonya, Lori, and Colleen, for every late-night phone call, crying-strategy session, and supportive text.

Hillary Frank and her staff at *The Longest Shortest Time*, who were the first people to really give me a microphone, and who edited those first stories together with such elegance.

Every Airbnb host who allowed me to hermit away in your space. The folks at Getaway and Breitenbush Hot Springs for creating environments custom-made for people with ADHD, who need to be as far removed from distractions as possible. The incredible Indralaya community and the caretakers of the land there, for stewarding the location I visit when I close my eyes and want to feel fully, completely home.

Our Lady J, for allowing me to tell a bit of her story. Willam and Jacob Tobia, for showing me that I didn't need a ghost writer after all. Precious Brady-Davis, for inspiring me to write a book. My friend Jody, for editing, ideating, and encouraging me along the way.

CT and Benji for yes, introducing us, but also showing up so fully to support us when Hailey and Lucas first came to live with us. Jersey and Loren, for being grown-up friends to our kids.

Heather, for being my best friend and primary support person for the majority of the time I have written about in this book. Your consistent love was vital to me for so many years, and I am so grateful for that.

Erin and Sam for being our first (and best!) parenting mentors. Matt Black for truly blazing the trail and showing me what my body was capable of.

Nick Adams at GLAAD, for teaching me how to tell my story effectively, for reminding me that I did not create transphobia, and for always being honest about how I can better serve my beloved trans community.

Lukas Soto (Ojibwe/Mapuche), for who you are in the world and for sharing your wisdom about why land acknowledgments matter and how to do them respectfully.

ABOUT THE AUTHOR

TRYSTAN REESE is an established thought leader, educator, and speaker on diversity, equity, and inclusion. He is a professionally trained anti-racism facilitator and curriculum designer, studying under Rev. Dr. Jamie Washington at the Social Justice Training Institute. Trystan has been an organizer in the trans community for nearly two decades and is on the frontlines of this generation's biggest fights for LGBTQ justice.

Trystan launched onto the global stage as "the pregnant man" in 2017 when his family's unique journey gained international media attention. He gave closing performances for The Moth Mainstage in Portland, Albuquerque, and Brooklyn. Trystan has partnered with many major media outlets, including CNN, NBC, *People*, and BuzzFeed, to bring his message of love and resilience to the mainstream.

The founder of Collaborate Consulting, Trystan provides customized training solutions for individuals, organizations, and communities interested in social justice. He has trained hundreds of medical providers on LGBTQ inclusion and has delivered keynotes at dozens of conferences and convenings.

He is married to his partner, Biff, and they live on the traditional homelands of the Clackamas, Chinook, Cowlitz, Kalapuya, Kathlamet, Multnomah, Wasco-Wishram, Tumwater, and many other Nations who made the Columbia Basin their home (also known as Portland, OR), with their three kids: Lucas, Hailey, and Leo. They are very happy.

collaborate.consulting | @biffandi